Neuropsychiatry of Traumatic Brain Injury

Editors

RICARDO E. JORGE
DAVID B. ARCINIEGAS

PSYCHIATRIC CLINICS
OF NORTH AMERICA

www.psych.theclinics.com

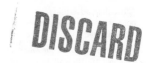

March 2014 • Volume 37 • Number 1

ELSEVIER

1600 John F. Kennedy Boulevard • Suite 1800 • Philadelphia, Pennsylvania, 19103-2899

http://www.theclinics.com

PSYCHIATRIC CLINICS OF NORTH AMERICA Volume 37, Number 1
March 2014 ISSN 0193-953X, ISBN-13: 978-0-323-28718-0

Editor: Joanne Husovski
Developmental Editor: Stephanie Carter

Psychiatric Clinics of North America (ISSN 0193-953X) is published quarterly by Elsevier Inc., 360 Park Avenue South, New York, NY 10010-1710. Months of issue are March, June, September, and December. Business and Editorial Offices: 1600 John F. Kennedy Blvd., Suite 1800, Philadelphia, PA 19103-2899. Periodicals postage paid at New York, NY and additional mailing offices. Subscription prices are $300.00 per year (US individuals), $546.00 per year (US institutions), $150.00 per year (US students/residents), $365.00 per year (Canadian individuals), $687.00 per year (Canadian Institutions), $455.00 per year (foreign individuals), $687.00 per year (foreign institutions), and $220.00 per year (international & Canadian students/residents). Foreign air speed delivery is included in all *Clinics'* subscription prices. All prices are subject to change without notice. **POSTMASTER:** Send address changes to *Psychiatric Clinics of North America*, Elsevier Health Sciences Division, Subscription Customer Service, 3251 Riverport Lane, Maryland Heights, MO 63043. Customer Service: 1-800-654-2452 (US). From outside the United States, call 1-314-447-8871. Fax: 1-314-447-8029. E-mail: journalscustomerservice-usa@elsevier.com (for print support) and journalsonlinesupport-usa@elsevier.com (for online support).

Reprints. For copies of 100 or more, of articles in this publication, please contact the Commercial Reprints Department, Elsevier Inc., 360 Park Avenue South, New York, New York 10010-1710. Tel.: 212-633-3874, Fax: 212-633-3820, E-mail: reprints@elsevier.com.

Psychiatric Clinics of North America is covered in *MEDLINE/PubMed (Index Medicus), Current Contents/Social and Behavioral Sciences, Social Science Citation Index, Embase/Excerpta Medica,* and PsycINFO.

Printed in the United States of America.

Contributors

EDITORS

RICARDO E. JORGE, MD
Professor of Psychiatry, Beth K. and Stuart C. Yudofsky Division of Neuropsychiatry, Baylor College of Medicine; Medical Director, TBI Center of Excellence, Michael E. DeBakey VA Medical Center, Houston, Texas

DAVID B. ARCINIEGAS, MD
Beth K. and Stuart C. Yudofsky Division of Neuropsychiatry, Chair in Brain Injury Medicine, Professor of Psychiatry, Neurology, and Physical Medicine & Rehabilitation, Menninger Department of Psychiatry and Behavioral Sciences, Baylor College of Medicine; Senior Scientist and Medical Director, Brain Injury Research Center, TIRR Memorial Hermann, Houston, Texas; Neuropsychiatry Service, Department of Psychiatry, University of Colorado School of Medicine, Aurora, Colorado

AUTHORS

IQBAL AHMED, MD
Faculty Psychiatrist, Tripler Army Medical Center and Clinical Professor of Psychiatry and Geriatric Medicine, University of Hawaii, Honolulu, Hawaii; Clinical Professor of Psychiatry, Uniformed Services of the Health Sciences, Bethesda, Maryland

DAVID B. ARCINIEGAS, MD
Beth K. and Stuart C. Yudofsky Division of Neuropsychiatry, Chair in Brain Injury Medicine, Professor of Psychiatry, Neurology, and Physical Medicine & Rehabilitation, Menninger Department of Psychiatry and Behavioral Sciences, Baylor College of Medicine; Senior Scientist and Medical Director, Brain Injury Research Center, TIRR Memorial Hermann, Houston, Texas; Neuropsychiatry Service, Department of Psychiatry, University of Colorado School of Medicine, Aurora, Colorado

NAZANIN H. BAHRAINI, PhD
Director of Education, Veteran Integrated Service Network (VISN) 19 Mental Illness Research Education and Clinical Center (MIRECC), Denver; Assistant Professor, Department of Psychiatry, School of Medicine, University of Colorado, Aurora, Colorado

LISA A. BRENNER, PhD, ABPP
Director, Veteran Integrated Service Network (VISN) 19 Mental Illness Research Education and Clinical Center (MIRECC), Denver; Associate Professor, Departments of Psychiatry, Neurology, and Physical Medicine and Rehabilitation, School of Medicine, University of Colorado, Aurora, Colorado

RYAN E. BRESHEARS, PhD
Director of Psychological Services, Wellstar Health System, Marietta; Adjunct Assistant Professor, Department of Counseling and Human Development, University of Georgia, Athens, Georgia

JERI E. FORSTER, PhD
Biostatistician, Veteran Integrated Service Network (VISN) 19 Mental Illness Research Education and Clinical Center (MIRECC), Denver; Assistant Professor, Department of Biostatistics & Informatics, Colorado School of Public Health, University of Colorado Denver, Denver, Colorado

DARYL E. FUJII, PhD
Staff Neuropsychologist, Veterans Affairs Pacific Island Health Care Services, Community Living Center, Honolulu, Hawaii

THERESA D. HERNÁNDEZ, PhD
Research Psychologist, Veteran Integrated Service Network (VISN) 19 Mental Illness Research Education and Clinical Center (MIRECC), Denver; Chair of the Department of Psychology and Neuroscience, University of Colorado, Boulder, Colorado

RICARDO E. JORGE, MD
Professor of Psychiatry, Beth K. and Stuart C. Yudofsky Division of Neuropsychiatry, Baylor College of Medicine; Medical Director, TBI Center of Excellence, Michael E. DeBakey VA Medical Center, Houston, Texas

HARVEY S. LEVIN, PhD
Director of Rehabilitation Research Center of Excellence, Michael E. DeBakey Veterans Affairs Medical Center; Professor, Departments of Psychiatry and Behavioral Sciences, Physical Medicine and Rehabilitation, Pediatrics, and Neurosurgery, Baylor College of Medicine, Houston, Texas

JEFFREY E. MAX, MBBCh
Professor, Department of Psychiatry, University of California, San Diego; Director, Neuropsychiatric Research, Rady Children's Hospital, San Diego, California

JAIME PAHISSA, MD
Department of Psychiatry, CEMIC University, Buenos Aires, Argentina

JENNIE L. PONSFORD, PhD
Professor of Neuropsychology, School of Psychological Sciences, Monash University; Director, Monash-Epworth Rehabilitation Research Centre, Epworth Hospital, Melbourne, Australia

AMANDA R. RABINOWITZ, PhD
Postdoctoral Fellow, Department of Neurosurgery, University of Pennsylvania School of Medicine, Philadelphia, Pennsylvania

ALEXANDRA L. SCHNEIDER, BA
Data Analyst, Veteran Integrated Service Network (VISN) 19 Mental Illness Research Education and Clinical Center (MIRECC), Denver, Colorado

JONATHAN M. SILVER, MD
Clinical Professor of Psychiatry, New York University School of Medicine, New York, New York

KELLY L. SINCLAIR, DPsych
Research Fellow, School of Psychological Sciences, Monash University; Monash-Epworth Rehabilitation Research Centre, Epworth Hospital, Melbourne, Australia

SERGIO E. STARKSTEIN, MD, PhD
School of Psychiatry and Clinical Neurosciences, University of Western Australia, Fremantle, Western Australia, Australia

HAL S. WORTZEL, MD
Veteran Integrated Service Network (19) Mental Illness Research Education and Clinical Center (MIRECC), Denver Veterans Medical Center, Denver; Neuropsychiatry Service, Department of Psychiatry, University of Colorado School of Medicine, Aurora, Colorado; Beth K. and Stuart C. Yudofsky Division of Neuropsychiatry, Menninger Department of Psychiatry and Behavioral Sciences, Baylor College of Medicine, Houston, Texas

Contents

Cognitive dysfunction is the leading cause of disability following traumatic brain injury (TBI). This article provides a review of the cognitive sequelae of TBI, with a focus on deficits of executive functioning and everyday thinking skills. The pathophysiology, assessment, and treatment of TBI-related cognitive problems are also discussed.

In this article, we examine the epidemiology and risk factors for the development of the most common mood disorders observed in the aftermath of TBI: depressive disorders and bipolar spectrum disorders. We describe the classification approach and diagnostic criteria proposed in the fifth edition of the Diagnostic and Statistical Manual for Mental Disorders. We also examine the differential diagnosis of post-TBI mood disorders and describe the mainstay of the evaluation process. Finally, we place a special emphasis on the analysis of the different therapeutic options and provide guidelines for the appropriate management of these conditions.

Emotional and behavioral dyscontrol are relatively common neuropsychiatric sequelae of traumatic brain injury and present substantial challenges to recovery and community participation. Among the most problematic and functionally disruptive of these types of behaviors are pathologic laughing and crying, affective lability, irritability, disinhibition, and aggression. Managing these problems effectively requires an understanding of their phenomenology, epidemiology, and clinical evaluation. This article reviews these issues and provides clinicians with brief and practical suggestions for the management of emotional and behavioral dyscontrol.

Given the upsurge of research in posttraumatic stress disorder (PTSD) and traumatic brain injury (TBI), much of which has focused on military samples who served in Iraq and Afghanistan, the purpose of this article is to review the literature published after September 11th, 2001 that addresses the epidemiology, pathophysiology, evaluation, and treatment of PTSD in the context of TBI.

than population base rates. Novel (postinjury onset) psychiatric disorders (NPD) are also common and complicate child function after injury. Novel disorders include personality change due to TBI, secondary attention-deficit/hyperactivity disorder, other disruptive behavior disorders, and internalizing disorders. This article reviews preinjury psychiatric disorders as well as biopsychosocial risk factors and treatments for NPD.

PSYCHIATRIC CLINICS OF NORTH AMERICA

FORTHCOMING ISSUES

June 2014
Obsessive Compulsive Disorder
Wayne Goodman, *Editor*

September 2014
Sexual Deviance: Assessment and
Treatment
John Bradford and
A.G. Ahmad, *Editors*

December 2014
Stress: What Physicians Need to Know
Daniel L. Kirsch and
Michel Woodbury, *Editors*

RECENT ISSUES

December 2013
Late Life Depression
W. Vaughn McCall, *Editor*

September 2013
Disaster Mental Health: Around the World
and Across Time
Craig L. Katz and
Anand Pandya, *Editors*

June 2013
Psychiatric Manifestations of Neurotoxins
Daniel E. Rusyniak and
Michael R. Dobbs, *Editors*

RELATED INTEREST

Neurologic Clinics
February 2014 (Vol. 32, No. 1)
Neuroimaging
Laszlo Mechtler, *Editor*

Preface

Neuropsychiatry of Traumatic Brain Injury

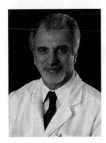 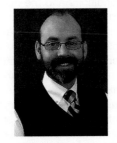

Ricardo E. Jorge, MD   David B. Arciniegas, MD
Editors

Traumatic brain injury (TBI) is a common and clinically important problem in North America: each year, more than 1.7 million individuals experience a TBI requiring hospital-based medical evaluation,[1] 1.6 to 3.8 million sustain injuries for which no immediate medical attention is sought,[2] 125,000 develop TBI-related disability,[3] and 3.2 million people live with chronic TBI-related disability.[4] The health and functional consequences of TBI are many and varied,[5] among the most challenging of which are neuropsychiatric problems,[6–9] including cognitive impairments, disorders of mood and affect, posttraumatic stress disorder, behavioral disturbances, and sleep disorders, among many others.[10,11]

The delimitation of neuropsychiatric disorders associated with TBI and the elucidation of the complex way in which these conditions overlap and interact are subjects of active investigation. Progress in this field is spurred by advances in basic and clinical neuroscience that are gradually unveiling how the structural and functional brain changes produced by TBI might influence the onset and clinical presentation of neuropsychiatric disorders. Certainly, a description of this body of research is an excellent focus of review. However, the need for psychiatric care among persons with TBI and their families is substantial[12–17] and this need too often goes unmet in American health care systems.[18–21] Consequently, this issue of *Psychiatric Clinics of North America* is intended to provide psychiatrists, psychologists, psychiatric nurses, social workers, and allied mental health clinicians with information that will help them meet this need. The selection of the themes as well as the format and content of the articles included in this volume were made with this priority in mind.

We invited a group of internationally renowned experts in the field of brain injury neuropsychiatry and neuropsychology to join us in providing nine concise and practical reviews addressing the most common and clinically challenging neuropsychiatric sequelae of TBI. Drs Rabinowitz and Levin describe the cognitive sequelae of TBI and emphasize the role of cognitive rehabilitation in the care of persons with TBI.

Psychiatr Clin N Am 37 (2014) xi–xv
http://dx.doi.org/10.1016/j.psc.2013.12.002
0193-953X/14/$ – see front matter

We provide a review of the evaluation and treatment of mood disorders after TBI, and one of us (D.A.) collaborated with Dr Wortzel to provide an overview of the phenomenology, evaluation, and treatment of disorders of emotional and behavioral dyscontrol experienced by persons with TBI. Drs Bahraini, Breshears, Hernández, Schneider, Forster, and Brenner follow with a review of TBI, postconcussive symptoms, and posttraumatic stress disorder in civilians, service members, and Veterans, emphasizing the distinct but interacting nature of these conditions and the need for their concurrent evaluation and management. Drs Ponsford and Sinclair's review focuses on posttraumatic sleep disturbances and fatigue; their work identifies these not only as specific clinical problems but also ones that complicate other posttraumatic neuropsychiatric conditions. Dr Silver describes the problem of persistent postconcussive symptoms and provides a master clinician's approach to the evaluation and management of persons with this challenging clinical presentation. Drs Starkstein and Pahissa describe the evaluation and management of the apathy syndrome among persons with TBI and Drs Fujii, Ahmed, and Fujii provide both conceptual and practical considerations of posttraumatic psychoses. Finally, Dr Max offers a concise overview of the neuropsychiatry of pediatric TBI.

These reviews focus principally on the evaluation and management of psychiatric problems occurring in the subacute and chronic periods after mild, moderate, or severe TBI. Each review includes a synopsis and key points that highlight concepts, assessment issues, and management approaches that readers may find useful in daily practice. These works highlight the typically rapid and complete recovery experienced by most persons with mild TBI,[22–25] while acknowledging that psychiatric symptoms may become complex and persistent challenges for a minority of persons with such injuries.[26–28] Opportunities to improve long-term neuropsychiatric and functional outcomes among persons with moderate or severe TBI also are identified and coupled with evidence-informed approaches that clinicians can use toward those ends.

Across these works, the authors consistently note the need to consider the interactions between preinjury (eg, age, gender, neurogenetic, developmental, psychiatric), injury-related (eg, injury type, severity, and location or locations, neuroendocrine, inflammatory, and metabolic alterations), and postinjury (eg, types and timings of interventions, social supports, other stressors) factors in the development of posttraumatic neuropsychiatric disturbances. This approach echoes and extends the direction offered by the British neurologist Sir Charles P. Symonds, MD, more than 75 years ago,[29] who said:

"The later effects of head injury can only be properly understood in light of a full psychiatric study of the individual patient, and in particular, his constitution. In other words, it is not only the kind of injury that matters, but the kind of head."

The authors of the present reviews also emphasize the importance of considering the differential diagnosis for posttraumatic neuropsychiatric disturbances among persons with TBI and directing treatment at comorbidities contributing to (or accounting for) neuropsychiatric symptoms. When appropriate, the authors address relevant changes in psychiatric nosology introduced in the fifth edition of the Diagnostic and Statistical Manual of Mental Disorders (DSM-5)[30] and emphasize the benefit of using both categorical and dimensional measures in the evaluation of persons with posttraumatic neuropsychiatric disturbances.

With regard to treatments, this set of authors also generally regards nonpharmacologic (ie, psychological, behavioral, environmental) interventions as first-line and symptom-targeted pharmacotherapies as adjunctive. We hope that these concise clinical reviews and the practical guidance they provide will be of value to clinicians and will facilitate their efforts to improve the lives of individuals and families affected by TBI.

This issue is a product of a large team whose collective efforts we must acknowledge here. We appreciate the contributions of our friends and colleagues whose articles comprise this issue of *Psychiatric Clinics of North America*, and we are grateful to our families for their encouragement and forbearance during the preparation of this volume. We also are deeply indebted to Joanne Husovski, Senior Editor, and Stephanie Carter, Developmental Editor, at Elsevier for inviting us to collaborate on the development of this issue and for guiding us through its production.

Ricardo E. Jorge, MD
Beth K. and Stuart C. Yudofsky Division of Neuropsychiatry
Baylor College of Medicine
TBI Center of Excellence
Michael E. DeBakey VA Medical Center

David B. Arciniegas, MD
Psychiatry, Neurology, and Physical Medicine and Rehabilitation
Baylor College of Medicine
Brain Injury Research
TIRR Memorial Hermann

E-mail addresses:
Ricardo.Jorge@bcm.edu (R.E. Jorge)
David.Arciniegas@bcm.edu (D.B. Arciniegas)

REFERENCES

1. Faul M, Xu L, Wald MM. Traumatic brain injury in the United States: emergency department visits, hospitalizations, and deaths 2002-2006. Atlanta (GA): National Center for Injury Control and Prevention, Centers for Disease Control and Prevention; 2010.
2. Langlois JA, Rutland-Brown W, Wald MM. The epidemiology and impact of traumatic brain injury: a brief overview. J Head Trauma Rehabil 2006;21(5):375–8.
3. Selassie AW, Zaloshnja E, Langlois JA, et al. Incidence of long-term disability following traumatic brain injury hospitalization, United States, 2003. J Head Trauma Rehabil 2008;23(2):123–31.
4. Zaloshnja E, Miller T, Langlois JA, et al. Prevalence of long-term disability from traumatic brain injury in the civilian population of the United States, 2005. J Head Trauma Rehabil 2008;23(6):394–400.
5. Zasler ND, Katz DI, Zafonte RD. Brain injury medicine: principles and practice. 2nd edition. New York: Demos Medical Publishing; 2013.
6. Kim E, Lauterbach EC, Reeve A, et al. Neuropsychiatric complications of traumatic brain injury: a critical review of the literature (a report by the ANPA Committee on Research). J Neuropsychiatry Clin Neurosci 2007;19(2):106–27.
7. Bhalerao SU, Geurtjens C, Thomas GR, et al. Understanding the neuropsychiatric consequences associated with significant traumatic brain injury. Brain Inj 2013; 27(7–8):767–74.
8. Arciniegas DB, Zasler ND, Vanderploeg RD, et al. Management of adults with traumatic brain injury. 1st edition. Washington, DC: American Psychiatric Publishing; 2013.

9. Bryant RA, O'Donnell ML, Creamer M, et al. The psychiatric sequelae of traumatic injury. Am J Psychiatry 2010;167(3):312–20.

10. Silver JM, McAllister TW, Yudofsky SC. Textbook of traumatic brain injury. 2nd edition. Arlington (VA): American Psychiatric Publishing; 2011.

11. Arciniegas DB, Zasler ND, Vanderploeg RD, et al. Management of adults with traumatic brain injury. Washington, DC: American Psychiatric Publishing; 2013.

12. Rotondi AJ, Sinkule J, Balzer K, et al. A qualitative needs assessment of persons who have experienced traumatic brain injury and their primary family caregivers. J Head Trauma Rehabil 2007;22(1):14–25.

13. Sayer NA, Cifu DX, McNamee S, et al. Rehabilitation needs of combat-injured service members admitted to the VA Polytrauma Rehabilitation Centers: the role of PM&R in the care of wounded warriors. PM R 2009;1(1):23–8.

14. McCarthy ML, Dikmen SS, Langlois JA, et al. Self-reported psychosocial health among adults with traumatic brain injury. Arch Phys Med Rehabil 2006;87(7): 953–61.

15. Corrigan JD, Whiteneck G, Mellick D. Perceived needs following traumatic brain injury. J Head Trauma Rehabil 2004;19(3):205–16.

16. Feeney TJ, Ylvisaker M, Rosen BH, et al. Community supports for individuals with challenging behavior after brain injury: an analysis of the New York state behavioral resource project. J Head Trauma Rehabil 2001;16(1):61–75.

17. Andelic N, Sigurdardottir S, Schanke AK, et al. Disability, physical health and mental health 1 year after traumatic brain injury. Disabil Rehabil 2010;32(13): 1122–31.

18. Brenner LA, Homaifar BY, Olson-Madden JH, et al. Prevalence and screening of traumatic brain injury among veterans seeking mental health services. J Head Trauma Rehabil 2013;28(1):21–30.

19. Olson-Madden JH, Brenner LA, Matarazzo BB, et al. Identification and treatment of TBI and co-occurring psychiatric symptoms among OEF/OIF/OND veterans seeking mental health services within the State of Colorado: establishing consensus for best practices. Community Ment Health J 2013;49(2):220–9.

20. Kurowski BG, Wade SL, Kirkwood MW, et al. Behavioral predictors of outpatient mental health service utilization within 6 months after traumatic brain injury in adolescents. PM R 2013.

21. Johnstone B, Nossaman LD, Schopp LH, et al. Distribution of services and supports for people with traumatic brain injury in rural and urban Missouri. J Rural Health 2002;18(1):109–17.

22. Carroll LJ, Cassidy JD, Peloso PM, et al. Prognosis for mild traumatic brain injury: results of the WHO Collaborating Centre Task Force on Mild Traumatic Brain Injury. J Rehabil Med 2004;(Suppl 43):84–105.

23. Department of Veterans Affairs and Department of Defense. VA/DoD Clinical Practice Guideline for Management of Concussion/Mild Traumatic Brain Injury. J Rehabil Res Dev 2009;46(6):CP1–68.

24. Rohling ML, Binder LM, Demakis GJ, et al. A meta-analysis of neuropsychological outcome after mild traumatic brain injury: re-analyses and reconsiderations of Binder, et al. (1997), Frencham et al. (2005), and Pertab et al. (2009). Clin Neuropsychol 2011;25(4):608–23.

25. Dikmen SS, Corrigan JD, Levin HS, et al. Cognitive outcome following traumatic brain injury. J Head Trauma Rehabil 2009;24(6):430–8.

26. Ruff RM, Camenzuli L, Mueller J. Miserable minority: emotional risk factors that influence the outcome of a mild traumatic brain injury. Brain Inj 1996;10(8): 551–65.

27. McCrea M, Iverson GL, McAllister TW, et al. An integrated review of recovery after mild traumatic brain injury (MTBI): implications for clinical management. Clin Neuropsychol 2009;23(8):1368–90.
28. Belanger HG, Spiegel E, Vanderploeg RD. Neuropsychological performance following a history of multiple self-reported concussions: a meta-analysis. J Int Neuropsychol Soc 2010;16(2):262–7.
29. Symonds CP. Mental disorder following head injury. Proc R Soc Med 1937;30(9): 1081–94.
30. American Psychiatric Association DSM-5 Task Force. Diagnostic and Statistical Manual of Mental Disorders: DSM-5. 5th edition. Washington, DC: American Psychiatric Association; 2013. p. xliv, 947.

Cognitive Sequelae of Traumatic Brain Injury

Amanda R. Rabinowitz, PhD[a],*, Harvey S. Levin, PhD[b]

KEYWORDS

- Traumatic brain injury • mTBI • Concussion • Executive functioning
- Neuropsychological assessment

KEY POINTS

- Cognitive deficits are a common consequence of acute traumatic brain injury (TBI), even at the lowest level of injury severity: concussion and mild TBI (mTBI). Approximately 65% of patients with moderate to severe TBI report long-term problems with cognitive functioning, and as many as 15% of patients with mTBI have persistent problems, which often include cognitive deficits.
- Deficit leads to disability when it interferes with patients' functional status (ie, their ability to perform their usual preinjury activities). Cognitive dysfunction is the leading cause of TBI-related disability, which affects approximately 43% of moderate to severe patients.
- Frontal lobe regions and their related circuitry are particularly vulnerable to TBI pathophysiology; and hence, executive deficits are common.
- Evaluation of cognitive functions should be routine in the assessment and treatment of postacute TBI. Referral to a neuropsychologist can provide a thorough profile of an individual patient's cognitive strengths and weaknesses, which may aid in setting goals for treatment, career and education planning, or provide information about independent functioning.
- Cognitive rehabilitation therapy (CRT) is a safe treatment option for patients with TBI with cognitive deficits; however, more methodologically rigorous research is needed to demonstrate its efficacy and identify which patients are most likely to respond.

INTRODUCTION

Traumatic brain injury (TBI) has a profound effect on injured individuals and their families. Cognitive deficits caused by TBI interfere with work, relationships, leisure, and

This research was supported by Mild Traumatic Brain Injury and Diffuse Axonal Injury. NINDS Grant P01 NS056202 awarded to Douglas Smith, MD, and Neurobehavioral Outcome of Head Injury in Children. NINDS Grant NS-21889 awarded to Gerri Hanten, PhD, and Harvey Levin, PhD.
[a] Department of Neurosurgery, University of Pennsylvania School of Medicine, 370 Stemmler Hall, Philadelphia, PA 19104, USA; [b] Michael E. DeBakey Veterans Affairs Medical Center, 2002 Holcombe Boulevard, Houston, TX 77030, USA; and Departments of Psychiatry and Behavioral Sciences, Physical Medicine and Rehabilitation, Pediatrics, and Neurosurgery, Baylor College of Medicine, 6560 Fannin #1144, Houston, TX 77030, USA
* Corresponding author.
E-mail address: rabinowitz.a@gmail.com

Psychiatr Clin N Am 37 (2014) 1–11
http://dx.doi.org/10.1016/j.psc.2013.11.004
psych.theclinics.com

Abbreviations	
TBI	Traumatic brain injury
PTA	Posttraumatic amnesia
mTBI	Mild traumatic brain injury
DAI	Diffuse axonal injury
DLPFC	Dorsolateral prefrontal cortex
DTI	Diffusion tensor imaging
FITBIR	Federal Interagency Traumatic Brain Injury Research
NIH	National Institutes of Health
CDEs	Common data elements
CRT	Cognitive rehabilitation therapy
GMT	Goal Management Training
IOM	Institute of Medicine

activities of daily living, exacting a personal and economic cost that is difficult to quantify.

The cognitive sequelae of TBI are determined by a number of injury-related variables, including TBI severity, complications, concomitant injuries to other body regions, and chronicity of the injury. Patient characteristics, such as age, preinjury neuropsychiatric status, and genotype also play a role. In addition, cognitive recovery from TBI also can be moderated by the quality of the postacute environment.

In this article, we review the cognitive sequelae of closed head injury in adults, with a focus on deficits of executive function and everyday decision making. Although animal models have made valuable contributions to knowledge of TBI, we focus on human studies for the sake of clinical relevance. First, we review the epidemiology and nature of cognitive changes following TBI. We also discuss the pathophysiology of TBI-related cognitive deficits, and review clinical assessment and treatment options.

EPIDEMIOLOGY OF COGNITIVE DYSFUNCTION FOLLOWING TBI
Short-Term Cognitive Impairment

Impaired consciousness and posttraumatic amnesia (PTA) are neurobehavioral hallmarks of acute TBI. According to consensus definitions, moderate and severe TBI are characterized by loss of consciousness for longer than 30 minutes and/or PTA persisting for at least 24 hours. PTA is the transitory period of disorientation, confusion, and amnesia following TBI which leaves a gap in memory. Patients in PTA also commonly experience disturbed sleep-wake cycle, decreased daytime arousal, agitation, affective lability, and perceptual disturbance.[1] In PTA, gross fluctuations in the severity of cognitive and behavioral symptoms are common. During this acute confusional state, patients require supervision at the mild end of the spectrum and hospitalization at the moderate to severe end of the spectrum. Contrastingly, mild TBI (mTBI) may occur with or without loss of consciousness and PTA.

Recovery on clinical outcome measures typically occurs within several days after uncomplicated sports-related mTBI in young adults, but the clinical course can be longer in patients with other injury etiologies (eg, motor vehicle crashes), preinjury risk factors, concomitant injuries to other body regions, or age older than 50 years.

In general, cognitive deficits associated with mTBI resolve fully within 3 to 6 months in approximately 80% to 85% of patients who sustain their first mTBI without the presence of a brain lesion on computed tomography or other intracranial complication.[2] Although there appears to be a subgroup of patients with mTBI with persistent cognitive complaints,[3,4] the precise prevalence and etiology of these sequelae remain unclear. Data from a recent, prospective cohort study suggest that approximately one-third of patients with mTBI continue to experience functional impairment (Glasgow Outcome Scale-Extended score $\leq$6) 3 months postinjury.[5]

Moderate and severe TBI are associated with more severe and persistent cognitive deficits, which can involve cognitive domains typically preserved in mild TBI, such as awareness, reasoning, language, visuospatial processing, and general intelligence.

Long-Term Cognitive Impairment

As many as 65% of patients with moderate to severe TBI report long-term problems with cognitive functioning.[6] Cognitive deficits cause disability when they interfere with a patient's ability to perform their usual roles at work or home. Epidemiologic research indicates that about 43% of moderate and severe TBI patients experience disability over periods of 6 months or longer, characterized by functional limitations, postinjury symptoms that limit activities, cognitive complaints, and/or mental health problems.[7] Nearly a quarter of patients with moderate to severe TBI fail to return to work in the year following their injury.[6] At their most extreme, TBI-related cognitive deficits can impair a patient's ability to perform activities of daily living, such as driving, meal preparation, and handling money. Although TBI can cause sensory and motor deficits, cognitive and behavioral changes are more closely associated with long-term disability.[8]

In general, the relationship between acute TBI severity and cognitive sequelae is approximately linear, with longer duration of impaired consciousness predicting greater extent of cognitive dysfunction.[9] However, heterogeneity in TBI pathology and patient characteristics also influence cognitive outcomes, complicating prediction of recovery. The cognitive domains that are most often affected by mild to moderate TBI include memory, attention, processing speed, and executive functioning and are mostly resolved within 3 to 6 months of injury.[2,10–12] However, it is possible that cognitive dysfunction in a subgroup of individuals is poorly characterized by effect-size estimates based on aggregate data.[13] Moderate to severe TBI is also associated with deficits in memory, attention, processing speed, and executive functioning, and additionally involves functions such as communication, visuospatial processing, intellectual ability, and awareness of deficit.[14–16]

Cognitive recovery after moderate to severe TBI has a steep trajectory in the first year followed by more gradual improvements during later years. Impairments are more likely to persist in patients with severe injuries, although some patients may exhibit neuropsychological recovery up to 5 years after injury.[17] Gains in cognitive performance after the first year are likely to be a function of new learning and development of compensatory strategies.[17] A summary of the acute and long-term cognitive sequelae of TBI is provided in **Table 1**.

DEFICITS OF EXECUTIVE FUNCTION AND EVERYDAY THINKING SKILLS

Executive functioning deficits are common following TBI, even among those with mild injuries. The term "executive function" describes a variety of high-order cognitive abilities predominantly subserved by regions in the prefrontal cortex and their circuitry. Deficits of the executive system threaten an individual's ability to engage successfully in independent goal-oriented behavior. These functions are critically important for quality of life, as they are implicated in job performance, social relationships, and both basic and instrumental activities of daily living.[18] Results of a recent study suggest that executive deficits are more predictive of functional disability than demographic and injury variables.[19] Both cognitive and behavioral functions fall under the general umbrella of executive functioning, and many of these can be affected by TBI.

| Table 1 | | |
| Acute and long-term cognitive sequelae of TBI by levels of severity | | |
	Mild TBI	Moderate-Severe TBI
Acute		
Loss of consciousness (min)	0–30	>30
Posttraumatic amnesia (h)	0–24	>24
Subacute and long-term		
Memory	Resolves rapidly within	Persists in ~65% of patients[8]
Attention	80%–85% patients[2,10–12]	Can include deficits of
Processing speed	May persist in ~15% of	awareness, reasoning,
Executive functions	patients[13]	language, visuospatial
		processing, and general
		intelligence[14–16]

- Cognitive executive functions
  - Memory acquisition and retrieval
  - Top-down control of attention
  - Planning
  - Judgment
  - Cognitive aspects of decision making
- Behavioral executive functions
  - Emotional aspects of decision making
  - Motivation
  - Impulsivity

Various investigators have conceptualized executive functions in a number of different ways. Characterizations tend to share in common the notion that the executive system involves distinct components, which are, at least to some extent, functionally and anatomically dissociable. Within an individual patient any number of these functional domains may be affected or spared. Nearly all characterizations of executive function include components describing the control and direction of lower level cognitive abilities, motivation, and self-monitoring. These functions influence many everyday cognitive tasks, including learning and memory, planning, decision making, and social behavior.[18,20]

Executive dysfunction can lead to apparent disruption of cognitive performance in other related domains, such as memory and top-down control of attention. Memory problems are a common complaint following TBI, but the nature of TBI-related memory difficulties is quite different from what is typically seen in Alzheimer disease or other amnestic memory disorders. Unlike an amnestic memory disorder, memory problems in TBI are not typically due to a deficit of memory storage; that is, patients with TBI generally retain the ability to recognize newly learned material. Rather, patients with TBI tend to have difficulties organizing new information for successful encoding and retrieval.[21,22] Because of disorganized memory encoding patients with TBI are more likely to attribute information to the wrong source (eg, a patient might misremember that a piece of information was told to him by his wife, when it was in fact relayed by his doctor). They are also more likely to conflate different pieces of information (eg, a patient might mistakenly conflate the appointment date for a doctor's appointment with the appointment time for a salon appointment).

Planning abilities are also depressed following TBI. Effective planning depends on an individual's ability to hold rules and conditions in mind using working memory, represent and keep track of available options, and forecast the consequences of each course of action. These skills are typically evaluated using tests that require the examinee to achieve a goal as efficiently as possible, while following a set of rules. Patients with TBI are more likely than uninjured individuals to violate the rules and take unnecessary steps in their execution of a task.[23] These types of difficulties translate to real-life problems, such as inefficiencies and errors on the job or at home. Instrumental activities of daily living, such as cooking, shopping, driving, and finance management, can be affected.

Judgment and decision making may also be impaired in moderate-to-severe TBI; however, these deficits are rare at the mild end of the TBI severity spectrum.[24] Human reasoning depends on both effortful cognitive operations and the automatic input from visceral or emotional states.[25] The somatic marker hypothesis has been put forth to explain the role of emotion in decision making. Decision-making typically involves the selection of an option among a set of choices (decision space). According to the somatic marker hypothesis, humans associate visceral and emotional states with each item in the decision space according to their prior experience with those options. Options associated with reward are emphasized, whereas those associated with negative outcomes are suppressed. These emotional inputs are integrated with rational analysis to produce a decision.[26] Changes in the neural mechanisms underlying visceral responses and their associations with positive and negative outcomes can impair an individual's ability to optimally adjust their behavior in the face of risks. Patients with moderate to severe TBI may exhibit deficits in the various aspects of decision making, such as impulsivity, risk adjustment, and rational choice. These impairments are related to neuroimaging abnormalities in the anatomic regions associated with each of those functions.[27]

The diminished capacity to initiate activity can be one of the most devastating consequences of a brain injury. Apathy is a condition characterized by reduced goal-directed activity and lowered motivation. Point-prevalence rates of apathy in patients with severe TBI range from 46% to 71%.[28] This is a serious problem, as it can lead to social withdrawal and neglect of important self-care activities. Across neurologic diseases, apathy is associated with a number of adverse outcomes, including decreased functional level, caregiver distress, and poor treatment response.[26] It is unclear whether apathy is the cause of these deleterious outcomes, or if apathy and negative outcomes are associated via a lurking variable, such as injury severity. Deficits in motivation and drive are more prevalent in severe TBI with focal lesions involving the right frontal lobe.[26]

Deficits of self-awareness and self-monitoring are also associated with severe TBI. As might be expected, these problems pose a serious challenge for rehabilitation and treatment. At its most severe, patients exhibit anosognosia, or the failure to recognize the existence of a disease or injury.[29] Impaired awareness can take on many forms in patients with TBI. Acutely, patients may be unaware that they have suffered an injury at all. Later in the clinical course, patients may be aware of their injury, but underestimate its impact on their ability to function.[30] Patients tend to have better awareness for physical (eg, hemiparesis) rather than cognitive deficits.[30]

Metacognition refers to the conscious awareness of one's cognitive abilities.[31] Metacognitive knowledge describes patients' general awareness of their cognitive abilities, which can be measured by evaluating the discrepancy between self-report of cognitive problems and actual neuropsychological performance. Emergent and anticipatory awareness during the execution of a cognitive task represent a different category of metacognitive skills. The ability to notice and respond to errors is an emergent form of awareness that allows an individual to modulate his or her approach to a task so as to optimize success. The ability to predict future performance is an anticipatory metacognitive skill that allows an individual to forecast his or her success and prepare for optimal performance.[32] Each of these metacognitive skills can be affected by TBI.

PATHOPHYSIOLOGY OF COGNITIVE DEFICITS FOLLOWING TBI

Closed head TBI occurs when the brain undergoes rapid acceleration-deceleration forces, which may involve blunt head impacts. However, rapid acceleration or deceleration of the head can occur without impact. The resultant biomechanical forces can include both translational (the head moving in a straight line with the brain's center of gravity) and rotational (the brain rotating around its center of gravity) accelerations. Although there is great heterogeneity in the biomechanical profile of TBI, there is a predominant injury profile that suggests the vulnerability of specific gray matter regions and white matter pathways. Contusions, or focal damage to the brain's tissue and vasculature structure, are most likely to occur in frontal and temporal regions where brain tissue is adjacent to the bony ridges and protuberances of the interior base of the skull.[33] Intracranial hemorrhage may occur, and represents an acute medical emergency. Diffuse axonal injury (DAI) refers to damage of the brain's white matter tracts, caused by sheering forces that result when the brain rotates within the skull.[34,35] Due to axon's viscoelastic properties, axonal damage is prevalent across levels of injury severity, and DAI is likely to be the principal pathologic substrate of long-term deficits associated with mTBI.[36,37]

Given the high prevalence of executive deficits in patients with TBI, it is not surprising that the frontal lobes and their related circuitry (eg, subcortical white matter, basal ganglia, and thalamus) are particularly vulnerable to TBI.[38] Working memory and planning deficits may be associated with the focal injury to the dorsolateral prefrontal cortex (DLPFC) or DAI affecting the projections between the lateral frontal and posterior regions.[39] Apathy has been associated with subcortical lesions and right hemisphere dysfunction.[40] Impaired awareness is characteristic of patients with focal frontal injury,[41] and the postinjury level of self-referential insight has been associated with the integrity of right dorsal prefrontal cortex.[42]

Decision making is a complex cognitive function, and Newcombe and colleagues[27] examined the diffusion tensor imaging (DTI) correlates of its component skills in patients with moderate to severe TBI. Deficits in risk adjustment were associated with abnormalities in subcortical structures, such as the thalamus, the dorsal striatum, and the caudate. Impulsivity was associated with abnormal DTI findings in the bilateral orbital frontal gyri, insula, and caudate, whereas impaired rational choice was related to changes in the bilateral DLPFC, the superior frontal gyri, and the right and ventromedial prefrontal cortex, ventral striatum, and hippocampus. This pattern of results suggests that the emotional components of decision making (ie, risk adjustment and impulse control) predominantly involve subcortical structures and the interplay between frontal and subcortical systems, whereas cognitive components of decision making, such as rational choice, rely heavily on the prefrontal cortex.

Focal structural abnormalities are infrequent on computed tomography within 24 hours after mTBI. However, advanced neuroimaging techniques have begun to elucidate the effects of mild brain injury. DTI is a neuroimaging technique that measures the diffusion of water in tissues, which has been used to evaluate the integrity of the brain's white matter. DTI studies of patients with mTBI corroborate findings from patients with more severe injuries, suggesting that frontal and temporal pathways are most vulnerable to traumatic damage.[37,43–45]

NEUROPSYCHOLOGICAL ASSESSMENT

Cognitive functioning should be assessed in any patient with TBI. Interviewing the patient and a caregiver is recommended because a subgroup of patients with severe TBI has poor awareness of the presence or extent of their cognitive deficits and behavioral sequelae. An interview can evaluate the accuracy of the patient's insight concerning their condition by asking them to appraise their memory for events and names of people from 1 day to another, plans for return to work or school, organization of activities, and relations with family members, colleagues, and friends. Patients' self-reported problems provide the clinician with information regarding the deficits causing greatest subjective distress. Behavioral observations during an interview also can provide valuable information regarding the patient's sustained concentration, ability to shift attention from one task to another, and vulnerability to distraction. Comparison of the patient's report with input from a relative or caregiver is informative, especially if the collateral source is interviewed separately from the patient.

To harmonize research across centers and facilitate comparison of clinical data obtained at different sites, the Federal Interagency Traumatic Brain Injury Research Task Force, including the National Institutes of Health, has published a list of recommended outcome measures for clinical TBI research, referred to as Common Data Elements (CDEs). The CDEs include core, basic, and supplemental cognitive tests commonly used in clinical practice.[46,47]

Referral to a clinical neuropsychologist provides a more in-depth evaluation using tests that have been developed to be reliable and valid measures of cognition, behavior, and self-reported symptoms. With reference data obtained from large samples of representative subjects in the general population, the results of neuropsychological assessment can be reported in percentiles or standard scores that reflect the severity of deficits and relatively preserved abilities. Clinical neuropsychologists could also recommend further rehabilitation and other treatment that is implicated by the pattern of findings. **Box 1** lists several of the tests that are widely used by neuropsychologists to assess memory, attention, processing speed, and executive function. The "CDE" designation in **Box 1** denotes that it was recommended by panels of neuropsychologists as a Common Data Element.[46,47] The CDE outcome measures have been used extensively in research on recovery from TBI; the reliability and validity of these measures are also established.

There is an extensive body of literature supporting the sensitivity of neuropsychological tests to TBI-related cognitive deficits.[2,10,12,48] Typical neuropsychological assessment of TBI includes tests of episodic memory, attention, cognitive processing speed, and executive functions, such as mental flexibility, planning, decision making, inhibitory control, and organization. Assessment of mild TBI also should include a measure of postconcussion symptoms. For patients with moderate to severe injuries, awareness and judgment should be evaluated to determine the patient's capacity to function independently. The results of a neuropsychological assessment provide information regarding a patient's cognitive areas of weakness and preserved strengths. Findings can be particularly useful when there are questions regarding occupational and education planning. A neuropsychologist may also recommend strategies to help the patient compensate for deficits.

TREATMENT

Rehabilitation is a broad health care field primarily concerned with reducing patients' disability and enabling their independent functioning following a disease or injury. Rehabilitation for a physical disability, such as paralysis, might include physical

---

Box 1
Standard neuropsychological test battery to assess cognitive functioning following TBI

Memory

    Rey Auditory Verbal Learning (CDE)/California Verbal Learning Test- II (CDE)

    Brief Visuospatial Memory Test-Revised (CDE)

Processing Speed

    Wechsler Adult Intelligence Scale-IV Processing Speed Index (CDE)

Executive Functioning and Decision Making

    Controlled Oral Word Association (CDE)

    Trail Making Test (Trails A and B) (CDE)

    Color Word Interference (CDE)

    Iowa Gambling Task

Everyday Executive Functioning

    Behavioral Report Inventory of Executive Functioning—Adult

Symptom Validity Assessment

    Test of Memory Malingering (TOMM) (CDE)

Abbreviation: CDE, Common Data Element.

---

exercises, assistive technology, and skill training, as well as social services. Cognitive rehabilitation therapy (CRT) is a term that describes treatments designed to improve patients' participation in cognitive demanding activities, either by restoring cognitive functions or teaching compensatory skills. Like physical rehabilitation treatments, CRTs might incorporate technologies and services that facilitate patients' reintegration into their preinjury lifestyle.

Specific CRTs have been designed to address problems with attention, communication, memory, and executive functioning. Goal management training (GMT) is an example of a CRT for the treatment of executive functioning deficits based on theories of goal processing and sustained attention. Its primary objective is to train patients to periodically pause their ongoing behavior to monitor performance and define goal hierarchies. Cues, such as audible tones, can serve as reminders to stop and monitor behavior. A recent controlled study showed that brain-injured patients who received GMT showed evidence of cognitive improvements on tests of attention and planning.[49] The Institute of Medicine recently assembled a Committee on CRTs for TBI. The committee reviewed the evidence in support of CRTs across levels of injury, phases of recovery, and cognitive domains. They noted methodological limitations in the extant research literature on CRTs, but nonetheless, supported the ongoing use of CRTs for ameliorating the cognitive sequelae of TBI.[50] Future studies should use randomized controlled designs to best evaluate existing CRTs and identify which patients stand to benefit most from these interventions.

SUMMARY

Cognitive deficits are common following TBI and contribute significantly to disability. The frontal lobes and their related circuitry are particularly vulnerable to traumatic damage; hence, executive dysfunction is prevalent. Impairments in executive dysfunction can profoundly impact patients' quality of life, as these cognitive skills are implicated in job performance, social relationships, and activities of daily living. A neuropsychological evaluation provides a comprehensive assessment of patients' cognitive strengths and weaknesses. Cognitive rehabilitation is an appropriate treatment option for patients with TBI with cognitive deficits; however, more methodologically rigorous research is needed to demonstrate its efficacy and identify which patients are most likely to respond.

REFERENCES

1. Nakase-Richardson R, Yablon SA, Sherer M. Prospective comparison of acute confusion severity with duration of post-traumatic amnesia in predicting employment outcome after traumatic brain injury. J Neurol Neurosurg Psychiatry 2007; 78(8):872–6.
2. Belanger HG, Vanderploeg RD. The neuropsychological impact of sports-related concussion: a meta-analysis. J Int Neuropsychol Soc 2005;11(4): 345–57.
3. Boake C, McCauley SR, Levin HS, et al. Diagnostic criteria for postconcussional syndrome after mild to moderate traumatic brain injury. J Neuropsychiatry Clin Neurosci 2005;17(3):350–6.
4. Røe C, Sveen U, Alvsåker K, et al. Post-concussion symptoms after mild traumatic brain injury: influence of demographic factors and injury severity in a 1-year cohort study. Disabil Rehabil 2009;31(15):1235–43.
5. McMahon P, Hricik A, Yue JK, et al. Symptomatology and functional outcome in mild traumatic brain injury: results from the prospective TRACK-TBI study. J Neurotrauma 2013. [Epub ahead of print].
6. Whiteneck GG, Gerhart KA, Cusick CP. Identifying environmental factors that influence the outcomes of people with traumatic brain injury. J Head Trauma Rehabil 2004;19(3):191–204.
7. Selassie AW, Zaloshnja E, Langlois JA, et al. Incidence of long-term disability following traumatic brain injury hospitalization, United States, 2003. J Head Trauma Rehabil 2008;23(2):123–31.
8. Consensus conference. Rehabilitation of persons with traumatic brain injury. NIH Consensus Development Panel on rehabilitation of persons with traumatic brain injury. JAMA 1999;282(10):974–83.
9. Dikmen SS, Machamer JE, Winn HR, et al. Neuropsychological outcome at 1-year post head injury. Neuropsychology 1995;9(1):80.
10. Carroll L, Cassidy JD, Peloso P, et al. Prognosis for mild traumatic brain injury: results of the WHO collaborating centre task force on mild traumatic brain injury. J Rehabil Med 2004;43(Suppl):84–105.
11. Frencham KA, Fox AM, Maybery MT. Neuropsychological studies of mild traumatic brain injury: a meta-analytic review of research since 1995. J Clin Exp Neuropsychol 2005;27(3):334–51.
12. Schretlen DJ, Shapiro AM. A quantitative review of the effects of traumatic brain injury on cognitive functioning. Int Rev Psychiatry 2003;15(4):341–9.
13. Bigler ED, Farrer TJ, Pertab JL, et al. Reaffirmed limitations of meta-analytic methods in the study of mild traumatic brain injury: a response to Rohling, et al. Clin Neuropsychol 2013;27(2):176–214.
14. Ruff RM, Cullum CM, Luerssen TG. Brain imaging and neuropsychological outcome in traumatic brain injury. Neuropsychological function and brain imaging. USA: Springer; 1989. p. 161–83.

15. Pagulayan KF, Temkin NR, Machamer JE, et al. The measurement and magnitude of awareness difficulties after traumatic brain injury: a longitudinal study. J Int Neuropsychol Soc 2007;13(4):561–70.
16. Ruff RM, Marshall L, Crouch J, et al. Predictors of outcome following severe head trauma: follow-up data from the traumatic coma data bank. Brain Inj 1993;7(2):101–11.
17. Corrigan JD. Consequences of traumatic brain injury for functioning in the community. In: Ragnarsson KT, editor. Report of the NIH consensus development conference on the rehabilitation of persons with traumatic brain injury. Bethesda, MD: US Department of Health and Human Services; 1999. p. 64–8.
18. Lezak MD, Howieson DB, Bigler ED, et al. Neuropsychological assessment. USA: OUP; 2012.
19. Spitz G, Ponsford JL, Rudzki D, et al. Association between cognitive performance and functional outcome following traumatic brain injury: a longitudinal multilevel examination. Neuropsychology 2012;26(5):604–12.
20. Stuss DT. New approaches to prefrontal lobe testing. In: Miller BL, Cummings JL, editors. The Human Frontal Lobes: Functions and disorders. New York: The Guilford Press; 2007. p. 292–305.
21. Dikmen SS, Corrigan JD, Levin HS, et al. Cognitive outcome following traumatic brain injury. J Head Trauma Rehabil 2009;24(6):430–8.
22. Stuss DT, Alexander MP. Executive functions and the frontal lobes: a conceptual view. Psychol Res 2000;63:289–98.
23. Shum D, Gill H, Banks M, et al. Planning ability following moderate to severe traumatic brain injury: performance on a 4-disk version of the Tower of London. Brain Impair 2009;10(03):320–4.
24. Levin HS, Wilde E, Troyanskaya M, et al. Diffusion tensor imaging of mild to moderate blast-related traumatic brain injury and its sequelae. J Neurotrauma 2010; 27(4):683–94.
25. Bechara A, Damasio H, Damasio AR. Emotion, decision making and the orbitofrontal cortex. Cereb Cortex 2000;10(3):295–307.
26. Damasio A. The somatic-marker hypothesis. Descartes' error: emotion, reason, and the human brain. New York: GP Putnam's Sons; 1994. p. 165–201.
27. Newcombe VF, Outtrim JG, Chatfield DA, et al. Parcellating the neuroanatomical basis of impaired decision-making in traumatic brain injury. Brain 2011; 134(Pt 3):759–68.
28. van Reekum R, Stuss DT, Ostrander L. Apathy: why care? J Neuropsychiatry Clin Neurosci 2005;17:7–19.
29. Giancino JT, Cicerone KD. Varieties of deficit unawarness after brain injury. J Head Trauma Rehabil 1998;13(5):1–15.
30. Sherer M, Boake C, Levin E, et al. Characteristics of impaired awareness after traumatic brain injury. J Int Neuropsychol Soc 1998;4:380–7.
31. Flavell JH. Metacognition and cognitive monitoring: a new area of cognitive-developmental inquiry. American Psychologist 1979;34(10):906–11.
32. O'Keefe F, Dockree PM, Moloney P, et al. Awareness of deficits in traumatic brain injury: a multidimensional approach to assessing metacognitive knowledge and online-awareness. J Int Neuropsychol Soc 2007;13:38–49.
33. Genarelli T, Grabau D, editors. Neuropathology of head injures. Seminars in Clinical Neuropsychiatry 1998;3(3):160–75.
34. Gennarelli TA, Thibault LE, Adams JH, et al. Diffuse axonal injury and traumatic coma in the primate. Ann Neurol 1982;12(6):564–74.

35. Smith DH, Meaney DF. Axonal damage in traumatic brain injury. Neuroscientist 2000;6(6):483–95.
36. Browne KD, Chen XH, Meaney DF, et al. Mild traumatic brain injury and diffuse axonal injury in swine. J Neurotrauma 2011;28(9):1747–55.
37. Wilde E, McCauley S, Hunter J, et al. Diffusion tensor imaging of acute mild traumatic brain injury in adolescents. Neurology 2008;70(12):948–55.
38. MacDonald BC, Flashman LA, Saykin AJ. Executive dysfunction following traumatic brain injury: neural substrates and treatment strategies. NeuroRehabilitation 2002;17:333–44.
39. Cicerone KD, Levin HS, Malec JF, et al. Cognitive rehabilitation interventions for executive function: moving from bench to bedside in patients with traumatic brain injury. J Cogn Neurosci 2006;18(7):1212–22.
40. Andersson S, Krogstad JM, Finest A. Apathy and depressed mood in acquired brain damage: relationship to lesion localization and psychophysiological reactivity. Psychol Med 1999;29:447–56.
41. Spikman JM, van der Naalt J. Indices of impaired self-awareness in traumatic brain injury patients with focal frontal lesions and executive deficits: implications for outcome measurement. J Neurotrauma 2010;27(7):1195–202.
42. Schmitz TW, Rowley HA, Kawahara TN, et al. Neural correlates of self-evaluative accuracy after traumatic brain injury. Neuropsychologia 2006;44(5):762–73.
43. Bigler ED, Bazarian JJ. Diffusion tensor imaging. Neurology 2010;74(8):626–7.
44. Mayer A, Ling J, Mannell M, et al. A prospective diffusion tensor imaging study in mild traumatic brain injury. Neurology 2010;74(8):643–50.
45. Niogi S, Mukherjee P, Ghajar J, et al. Extent of microstructural white matter injury in postconcussive syndrome correlates with impaired cognitive reaction time: a 3T diffusion tensor imaging study of mild traumatic brain injury. AJNR Am J Neuroradiol 2008;29(5):967–73.
46. Wilde EA, Whiteneck GG, Bogner J, et al. Recommendations for the use of common outcome measures in traumatic brain injury research. Arch Phys Med Rehabil 2010;91(11):1650–60.
47. Hicks R, Giacino J, Harrison-Felix C, et al. Progress in developing common data elements for traumatic brain injury research: version two—the end of the beginning. J Neurotrauma 2013;30(22):1852–61.
48. Iverson GL. Outcome from mild traumatic brain injury. Curr Opin Psychiatry 2005;18(3):301.
49. Levine B, Schweizer TA, O'Connor C, et al. Rehabilitation of executive functioning in patients with frontal lobe brain damage with goal management training. Front Hum Neurosci 2011;5:9.
50. Committee on Cognitive Rehabilitation Therapy for Traumatic Brain Injury. Cognitive rehabilitation therapy for traumatic brain injury: evaluating the evidence. Washington, DC: Institute of Medicine; 2011.

Mood Disorders After TBI

Ricardo E. Jorge, MD[a,b,]*, David B. Arciniegas, MD[b,c]

KEYWORDS

• Traumatic brain injury • Mood disorders • Depressive disorders

KEY POINTS

• Depressive disorders are the most common neuropsychiatric sequels of traumatic brain injury (TBI). Mania, hypomania, and mixed mood states are less frequent but serious complications of TBI. In many respects, the evaluation and management of these conditions is similar to that provided to persons with primary (idiopathic) mood disorders.
• Mood disorders are highly comorbid with anxiety, substance misuse, and other behavioral alterations like impulsivity and aggression. Furthermore, once developed, they may have a chronic and refractory course.
• The functional repercussion of these disorders is huge, affecting the rehabilitation process as well as the long-term outcome of patients with TBI.
• Currently treatment options are, in a great part, dictated by expert opinion rather than by rigorous, adequately designed, and sufficiently large studies.

INTRODUCTION

Disorders of mood are common consequences of traumatic brain injury (TBI). The pathophysiology of mood disorders involves the interaction of factors that precede trauma (eg, genetic vulnerability and previous psychiatric history), factors that pertain to the traumatic injury itself (eg, type, extent, and location of brain damage), and factors that influence the recovery process (eg, family and social support). In some cases, especially in the early period following TBI, mood disturbance may reflect the effects

Support for this work was provided by the Veterans Health Administration's Traumatic Brain Injury Center of Excellence at the Michael E. DeBakey Veterans Affairs Medical Center, the National Institutes of Health grants RO1MH53592 and RO1 MH65134 01 (R.E. Jorge); the National Institute on Disability and Rehabilitation Research (NIDRR) grants H133A120020 and H133A130047 (D.B. Arciniegas). The content is solely the responsibility of the authors and does not necessarily represent the official views of the Department of Veterans Affairs or NIDRR.
[a] Mental Health Care Line, Michael E. DeBakey Veterans Affairs Medical Center, Menninger Department of Psychiatry and Behavioral Sciences, One Baylor Plaza, BCM 350, Houston, TX 77030, USA; [b] Beth K. and Stuart C. Yudofsky Division of Neuropsychiatry, Menninger Department of Psychiatry and Behavioral Sciences, Baylor College of Medicine, One Baylor Plaza, BCM 350, Houston, TX 77030, USA; [c] Brain Injury Research Center, TIRR Memorial Hermann, Menninger Department of Psychiatry and Behavioral Sciences, One Baylor Plaza, BCM 350, Houston, TX 77030, USA
* Corresponding author. One Baylor Plaza, BCM350, Houston, TX 77030.
E-mail address: jorge@bcm.edu

Psychiatr Clin N Am 37 (2014) 13–29
http://dx.doi.org/10.1016/j.psc.2013.11.005
0193-953X/14/$ – see front matter Published by Elsevier Inc.

Abbreviations	
BDI	Beck Depression Inventory
BDNF	Brain-derived neurotrophic factor
CBT	Cognitive behavioral therapy
CYP450	Cytochrome P450
DBS	Deep brain stimulation
DRO	Differential Reinforcement of Other Behavior
DTI	Diffusion tensor imaging
ECT	Electroconvulsive therapy
fMRI	Functional MRI
HAM-D	Hamilton Depression Scale
HMRS	Proton magnetic resonance spectroscopy
MAOIs	Monoamine oxidase inhibitors
MTHFR	Methylene tetrahydrofolate reductase
NOS	Not otherwise specified
PET	Positron emission tomography
PTSD	Post-traumatic stress disorder
rTMS	Repetitive transcranial magnetic stimulation
SSRIs	Selective serotonin reuptake inhibitors
TBI	Traumatic brain injury
TCAs	Tricyclic antidepressants
tDCS	Transcranial direct current stimulation
VNS	Vagal nerve stimulation

of neurotrauma on the distributed neural networks that generate and regulate emotion.[1] In some cases, especially those in which depressive disorders develop in the late postinjury period, psychological and social factors appear to be etiologically important.[1,2]

Mood disorders occur in the context of significant deficits in cognitive and emotional processing that may result from TBI. Individuals are challenged by deficits of which, in some cases, they are only partially aware. Consequently, life stressors increase and, in many cases, social support is reduced. These changes may lead to a disturbed and poorly integrated self-representation as well as to dysfunctional interpersonal relationships that increase the subjects' vulnerability to develop an affective episode. The high frequency and functional importance of disorders of mood among persons with TBI makes this an important topic for clinicians to understand.

DEPRESSIVE DISORDERS
Epidemiology

Depressive disorders develop commonly among persons with TBI, with estimated frequencies ranging from 6% to 77%.[3] Within this range, most experts on this subject accept an estimated first-year post-TBI depression frequency in the range of 25% to 50%[3,4] and lifetime rates of 26% to 64%.[5,6] The variability in the reported frequency of depressive disorders is related to the heterogeneity of the study groups as well as to the instruments used to ascertain a diagnosis of depression. In fact, many of the aforementioned studies have used arbitrary cutoffs in depression scales rather than conducting structured interviews and using accepted diagnostic criteria. We have studied the frequency and clinical correlates of depressive disorders occurring during the first year after TBI in 2 independent samples of patients with TBI recruited from an urban population in Maryland and a mostly rural population in Iowa. Depression diagnosis was made using a semistructured interview and the *Diagnostic and Statistical Manual of Mental Disorders* (DSM) nomenclature. In our studies, the frequency of major depression was 42% and 32%, respectively. Of note, depressive disorders were significantly more frequent among patients with TBI than in a control group of patients with orthopedic injuries. This suggests that the pathologic processes associated with TBI constitute an important contributing factor to the development of mood disorders.[7,8]

In our experience, depressive disorders following TBI were significantly associated with the presence of anxiety disorders. Approximately three-quarters of patients with depression had a coexistent anxiety disorder[8]; this finding was replicated in a recent prospective study that used a similar methodology.[9] In addition, major depression was associated with the occurrence of aggressive behavior[10] that, as expected, contributed to the deleterious effects of depression on community reintegration.

More recently, a study of 559 adults with complicated mild to severe TBI found that approximately half of patients (53.1%) developed major depression during the first year after TBI. Consistent with previous studies, major depression was frequently associated with significant anxiety, a history of affective illness, and a history of substance misuse.[11]

Although the risk of developing depression is generally regarded as being highest in the first postinjury year, the risk of this condition remains increased even decades after TBI. Hart and colleagues[12] analyzed the course of depressive disorders in the second year after TBI in a large sample (n = 1089) of subjects enrolled in the Traumatic Brain Injury Model Systems database. Approximately a fourth of patients who were not depressed during the first year following TBI developed depressive disorders during the second year. In addition, approximately two-thirds of subjects who were depressed during the first year after TBI continued to show significant depressive symptoms during the second year of follow-up.[12] Consistent with these observations in the early years after TBI, Koponen and colleagues[5] reported that major depression had a lifetime prevalence of 26.7% in a group of 60 patients with TBI followed for an average of 30 years.

Risk Factors

Genetic, demographic, developmental, and psychosocial factors, as well as their complex interactions, influence the risk of depression following TBI. There are no consistent data regarding the effect of age on the onset of mood disorders, particularly depression. Although some studies suggest that the frequency of psychiatric disorders and depression is greater among younger patients,[2,13] other investigators reported that depression is significantly more common in elderly patients.[14] A recent study reported a higher frequency of depressive symptoms in women than in men during the first 6 months after TBI.[15] However, there were no persistent gender differences in this study group at 1 year postinjury, and the mechanisms of early differences were not identified in this work. The issue of whether there are gender differences in depression following TBI remains unresolved, with a more recent study by our group finding no such effect.[8,16]

The literature investigating the effect of genetic factors for the development of depressive disorders after TBI is relatively scarce. A recent study examined the association between APOE-epsilon4 genotype and psychiatric disorders among 60 patients assessed an average of 30 years after severe TBI.[17] Cognitive disorders were significantly more common with the presence of APOE-epsilon4. The frequency of mood disorders, however, did not differ between patients with or without APOE-epsilon4 allele.

Polymorphisms in genes coding for proteins involved in the regulation of monoaminergic systems and of the hypothalamus-pituitary-adrenal axis (eg, 5HTT-P, tryptophan hydroxylase, MAO, COMT, FKBP5) and the interactions between genetic polymorphisms and environmental influences[18] might play a role in the likelihood of developing mood disorders.[19–28] Unfortunately, the effect of these factors on the psychiatric consequences of TBI has not been extensively studied and the effect sizes of those that have been identified are modest. Genetic polymorphisms modulating central dopaminergic pathways can affect prefrontal function following TBI[29,30]; however, it is not known if they have an effect on depressive disorders. Although a recent study failed to demonstrate an association between 5HTT polymorphisms and depression following TBI,[31] response to citalopram in this population is influenced by genotype, with adverse treatment effects occurring more frequently among persons with specific 5HTT polymorphisms and favorable treatment response predicted by the C-(677) T polymorphism of the methylene tetrahydrofolate reductase (MTHFR) gene and the val66met polymorphism of the brain-derived neurotrophic factor (BDNF) gene.[32]

Early psychosocial adversity (eg, history of physical or sexual abuse), life stress, and limited social support are also well-recognized risk factors for the development of psychiatric illness.[33,34] These factors have not been extensively studied among TBI populations. We found, however, that personal history of mood and anxiety disorders and previous poor social functioning are associated with the occurrence of major depression in the aftermath of TBI.[8,35] Furthermore, Fann and colleagues[36] observed that the risk of psychiatric illness is highest shortly after injury in persons with no psychiatric history, was unrelated to the severity of TBI, and appeared to increase in subsequent years in persons with previous psychiatric disorders.[36] This suggests that the effect of different risk factors varies over time and that psychosocial factors might be more relevant in the chronic stages of TBI.

Alcohol misuse is a significant risk factor for TBI, particularly when the latter occurs as a consequence of motor vehicle accidents or assault. We recently examined the relationship between alcohol misuse and the frequency of mood disorders among a group of 158 patients followed for a year after TBI. Of the 55 patients with TBI with a history of alcohol misuse, 33 (60%) developed a mood disorder during the first year of follow-up compared with 38 (36.9%) of 103 patients without a history of alcohol misuse.[37] Furthermore, three-quarters of patients who abused alcohol in the year after their TBI had a coexistent mood disorder.[37]

Diagnostic Assessment

Depressive disorders imply a pervasive and sustained alteration of emotion and affect that fundamentally alters one's way of being-in-the-world. As such, it impacts function in a wide variety of areas ranging from cognition to occupational performance and quality of life. The pervasive and, for many patients, recurrent nature of this alteration is essential for current classification schemes and helps to differentiate these disorders from other common emotional disorders among persons with TBI, especially the transient (ie, moment-to-moment) disturbances of emotional expression and experience that occur in this population, including emotional (or affective) lability and pathologic laughter and crying (or pseudobulbar affect).

During the past 2 decades, investigators strived to categorize psychiatric disturbances occurring after TBI within a common and reliable framework established by the DSM nomenclature. Standard diagnostic criteria for depression are appropriately applied to the diagnosis of depression among persons with TBI.[1] Overall, following the recently introduced DSM-V revision, depressive disorders associated with TBI are categorized as Mood Disorder Due to Another Medical Condition (TBI) with the following subtypes: (1) with major depressivelike episode (if the full criteria for a major depressive episode are met), (2) with depressive features (prominent depressed mood but full criteria for a major depressive episode are not met), and (3) with mixed features (when the predominant depressed mood coexists with maniclike symptoms).

Among patients with a preexisting mood disorder or whose depression develops in the late postinjury period, it may be more difficult to establish confidently that the depressive episode is a direct physiologic consequence of TBI. In such circumstances, a conservative approach is to indicate a diagnosis of depressive disorder not otherwise specified (NOS) and to regard TBI as an important and a possibly treatment-informing comorbidity rather than as a critical etiologic factor.

Structured or semistructured psychiatric interviews are useful to elicit a diagnosis of depression (and other psychiatric disorders) after TBI.[38,39] After establishing a categorical diagnosis of depression, symptom severity may be assessed using scales that are valid and reliable in this population. Particularly useful scales include the Beck Depression Inventory (BDI),[40] Hamilton Depression Scale (HAM-D),[7] Neurobehavioral Functioning Inventory Depression Scale,[41] or the Center for Epidemiologic Scales for Depression.[38] Clinician-administered scales offer advantages over self-report instruments, particularly among persons with limited insight due to TBI. Administration at the initial assessment and serially during the course of treatment provides information regarding the efficacy of interventions and may serve as an educational tool during psychotherapy.

Differential Diagnosis

The differential diagnosis of post-TBI depressive disorders includes, but is not limited to, delirium-associated mood disturbances, substance-related mood disturbances (including those related to substance intoxications, withdrawals, or medication induced), adjustment disorder with depressed and or anxious mood, pathologic laughter and crying, posttraumatic stress disorder (PTSD), posttraumatic apathy, personality change due to a general medical condition (especially labile type), and pre-TBI depressive disorders.

Pre-TBI mood (and especially depressive) disorders are common among persons with TBI[6,42] and must be included in the differential of any post-TBI depressive disorder. When such disorders are part of the pre-TBI history, it may not be possible to assert the role of TBI in the development and maintenance of postinjury depressive disorders. In these cases, it is important to observe if there has been a significant change in the clinical presentation of the current episode compared with the ones that occurred in the past (eg, the occurrence of prominent aggression or significant cognitive alterations) that might point to the relevance of the incident structural or functional brain damage.

Depressive symptoms may develop during posttraumatic delirium or along a substance withdrawal syndrome. These symptoms are usually evident as such rather than forming part of a depressive syndrome by virtue of the co-occurrence of other symptoms (eg, deficits in attention, fluctuating course, or autonomic instability) related to the pathophysiology of delirium. They tend to be labile and resolve in concert with the medical conditions underlying them. Medication-induced depressive symptoms are often more challenging to identify as such and, when suspected, tapering or discontinuing potentially causative medication is appropriate.

Adjustment disorders are related to the occurrence of a life stressor (eg, a motor vehicle accident), develop within 3 months of that stressor, and comprise a host of depressive and anxiety symptoms that are more transient and less severe than those observed in depressive disorders. In addition, they have significantly less impact on occupational and social functioning.

Apathy is frequently observed among patients with TBI, particularly those with more severe injuries, and may be mistaken for, or comorbid with, depression.[3,43] Apathy is a syndrome of diminished goal-directed behavior (as manifested by lack of effort, initiative, and productivity), cognition (as manifested by decreased interests, lack of plans and goals, and lack of concern about one's own health or functional status), and emotion (as manifested by flat affect, emotional indifference, and restricted responses to important life events).[44] Apathy is distinguished from depression by virtue of the absence of the core psychological symptoms of depression (ie, the apathetic patient is better described as "emotionally neutral" or "emotionally absent" than as one experiencing persistent and excessive sadness that negatively valences and distorts appraisal of the self, world, and future).

PTSD is also within the differential diagnosis for depression after TBI, and often these conditions coexist in the same individual. The presence of PTSD is suggested by reexperiences of the trauma through flashbacks or vivid nightmares, avoidance of circumstances related to the trauma, and emotional withdrawal or blunting. As the treatment for comorbid PTSD and depression differs from the treatment of depression alone, identification of this comorbidity is essential.

Pathologic laughter and crying, also called pseudobulbar affect, is in the differential diagnosis for depression among persons with TBI. It is characterized by the presence of stereotyped, sudden and uncontrollable affective outbursts (eg, crying or laughing). These emotional displays may occur spontaneously or may be triggered by minor stimuli. This condition lacks the pervasive alteration of mood, as well as the specific vegetative symptoms associated with a depressive episode.

Ancillary Studies

Physical examination, including a complete neurologic examination, is a requisite element of the initial evaluation along with conventional radiological procedures such as brain computed tomography scans or, in certain cases, magnetic resonance imaging (MRI) of the brain. Other neuroimaging techniques, such as quantitative MRI, diffusion tensor imaging, proton magnetic resonance spectroscopy, functional MRI (fMRI), and positron emission tomography, are increasing our understanding of the neurobiological bases of behavioral disorders among persons with TBI. However, these sophisticated research-based techniques require further validation before they can be routinely used in clinical and forensic settings. Quantitative electroencephalogram (EEG) and more complex electrophysiological responses may be relevant to the study of depression among persons with TBI[45,46] but have not been incorporated to clinical practice. If the history or examination suggests endocrine or diagnostically relevant physical conditions, then performing problem-focused laboratory studies are appropriate.[47] In light of the relatively high frequency of neuroendocrine abnormalities in this population,[48] screening for thyroid and growth hormone dysfunction is encouraged as part of the pretreatment depression evaluation. The American Psychiatric Association also suggests that physicians consider screening persons with depression for human immunodeficiency virus infections,[47] and encourages pretreatment urine and/or serum toxicology screening for alcohol and other substances of abuse.

Psychotherapy

Education regarding TBI and recovery expectations, reassurance, and frequent support is recommended as a part of all treatment plans for persons with these disorders.[49,50] Cognitive behavioral therapy may decrease depressive, anxious, and anger symptoms, as well as improve problem-solving skills, self-esteem, and psychosocial functioning following TBI.[51,52] Behavioral interventions, such as the Differential Reinforcement of Other Behavior may successfully reduce the frequency of problematic behavior.[53] In addition, psychotherapy groups implemented in postacute rehabilitation settings may focus on treatment of substance abuse and anger management through education, social support, and development of interpersonal skills.[54] More recently, Bell and colleagues[55] demonstrated the feasibility of using the telephone as a means of providing education and psychotherapeutic support during the first year after moderate to severe TBI.[55] Furthermore, in a recent study of 132 children with TBI, a Web-based counselor-assisted problem-solving intervention was shown to be efficacious to improve behavioral outcomes, including emotional well-being as rated by their primary caregivers.[56]

Peer support programs for persons with TBI and their families increase their knowledge about TBI, enhance coping with depression, and improve quality of life.[57] Attending to the psychological needs of spouses, families, and caregivers of persons with TBI is also important; post-TBI depression is strongly associated with significant family dysfunction[58] and depression is common among caregivers of persons with TBI.[59] Helping family members develop problem-solving and behavioral coping strategies also appears to decrease the severity of depression in the family member with TBI.[60] Engaging both the patient and their family members therefore is essential in the treatment of depression following TBI.

Pharmacotherapy

In general, the medications used to treat idiopathic depressive disorders are useful for the treatment of depression among persons with TBI. As with any medication intervention, clinicians are encouraged to refer to the product information sheet provided by the drug manufacturer for warnings and special considerations relevant to TBI, as well as for information on side effects, drug-drug interactions, treatment risks, and treatment contraindications before prescribing these or any other medications.

The selective serotonin reuptake inhibitors (SSRIs) and tricyclic antidepressants (TCAs) may improve depression following TBI.[61] Effective treatment of post-TBI depression with SSRIs also reduces comorbid irritability and aggression,[62] as well as the number and perceived severity of co-occurring somatic and cognitive symptoms.[63,64]

Concerns about both the tolerability and effectiveness of TCAs in this population lead most experts to regard them as second-line pharmacotherapies for depression after TBI and to recommend SSRIs as the first-line agents for this purpose. Among the SSRIs, sertraline and citalopram are favored in light of their beneficial effects, relatively limited side effects, and short half-lives. The use of other SSRIs, especially fluoxetine and paroxetine, is limited by their relatively greater potential for adverse effects and drug-drug interactions. For example, fluoxetine is a robust inhibitor of cytochrome P450 (CYP450) enzymes 2D6, 2C19, and 3A and is associated with problematic drug-drug interactions when coadministered with a substrate, inhibitor, or inducer of these enzymes. Paroxetine also is potent inhibitor of CYP450 2D6 and 2C19 and its significant anticholinergic effects increase the risk of treatment-related cognitive dysfunction even among healthy adults.[65] These issues limit enthusiasm for the use of fluoxetine or paroxetine to treat depression among persons with TBI.

Methylphenidate also has been compared to sertraline and placebo in a small double-blind, parallel-group study.[66] Both agents improved depression and methylphenidate, but not sertraline, also improved neuropsychological performance. Gualtieri and Evans[67] also observed similar methylphenidate-induced benefits on depression after TBI. Although methylphenidate would be an uncommon first-line intervention for depression after TBI in an outpatient setting, it may be useful for this purpose in an inpatient (including acute rehabilitation) setting or when a rapid therapeutic response is required. Early positive responses to methylphenidate in such circumstances are generally followed by a transition to maintenance therapy with an SSRI. Methylphenidate and other stimulants, including dextroamphetamine, also are used commonly to augment partial responses to SSRIs, especially when cognitive impairments and/or fatigue are residual symptoms during treatment with conventional antidepressants.

The efficacy and tolerability of other antidepressants, including the serotonin-norepinephrine reuptake inhibitors, bupropion, and the monoamine oxidase inhibitors (MAOIs), for the treatment of depression among persons with TBI are not well established. Many of these agents are used commonly in clinical practice and, in general, they appear to be similar to the SSRIs with respect to their benefits and adverse effects. However, using MAOIs is discouraged among persons with cognitive or other neurobehavioral impairments likely to reduced adherence to their dietary restrictions. Bupropion also is of concern in light of it propensity for lowering seizure threshold. This risk is greatest with the immediate-release form of bupropion.[68] Accordingly, using the sustained-release form of bupropion is prudent in this population and maintaining heightened vigilance for treatment-related seizures during treatment initiation and dose escalation is essential.

Amantadine, a drug with complex pharmacologic effects on glutamatergic, dopaminergic, and cholinergic systems might be of some use for the treatment of motivational deficits[69,70] and has shown beneficial to hasten recovery of patients with severe TBI and posttraumatic disorders of consciousness.[71] However, there are no data demonstrating a specific beneficial effect of amantadine on depression among persons with TBI.

Electroconvulsive Therapy and Brain Stimulation Techniques

Electroconvulsive therapy (ECT) may be used to treat of depression among persons with TBI who fail to respond to other interventions. When ECT is used for the treatment of posttraumatic depression, we recommend treatment with the lowest possible energy levels that will generate a seizure of adequate duration (greater than 20 seconds), using pulsatile currents, increased spacing of treatments (2 to 5 days between treatments), and fewer treatments in an entire course (ie, 4 to 6). If the patient also suffers from significant cognitive (especially memory) impairments due to TBI, nondominant unilateral ECT is the preferred technique.

Repetitive transcranial magnetic stimulation (rTMS) and transcranial direct current stimulation (tDCS) have not been rigorously studied in TBI populations. However, given that patients with TBI are more vulnerable to develop seizures in both the acute and chronic stages of their illness, tDCS and, alternatively, low-frequency rTMS, appear to be more suitable options to treat depressive disorders due to TBI.[72]

Vagal nerve stimulation and even deep brain stimulation of the ventral cingulate cortex also might be considered as a therapeutic option in an individual with unusually severe, treatment-refractory, and disabling symptoms. However, the use of this intervention among persons with depression following TBI also has not been studied specifically.

MANIC, HYPOMANIC, AND MIXED DISORDERS
Epidemiology

Bipolar and related disorders are relatively uncommon consequences of TBI.[73] Estimated frequencies of secondary mania (ie, an early post-TBI manic, hypomanic, or mixed episode that is unequivocally related to neurotrauma, usually involving right ventral frontal and/or basotemporal injury) range from 1.7% to 9.0%.[73,74] Clinical experience among rehabilitation specialists working in nonpsychiatric settings suggests that this condition occurs at a low frequency. In our studies, the frequency of bipolar and related mood episodes among the patients with TBI was 9.0%[75] and 6.5%[75] in Maryland and Iowa; these frequencies are based on relatively small samples (66 and 91 patients, respectively, in these studies). The episodes were short-lasting (ie, average duration of approximately 2 months), often involved mixed mood states, and associated with other externalizing features, such as aggression and substance misuse.[75] In these patients, mood symptoms not infrequently persisted for as long as 6 months despite resolution of other cognitive, behavioral, and vegetative manic symptoms.

The estimated lifetime relative risk for bipolar and related disorders after TBI ranges from 1.1 (in a sample of more than 5000 community-dwelling individuals interviewed in the Epidemiologic Catchment Area study),[73] a level of risk not statistically different than that of the general population, to 5.0 (in a review of 5 studies comprising 354 clinical subjects).[74] These estimates are influenced strongly by sample sizes, selection biases, and diagnostic ascertainment issues. Unfortunately, there are no studies that had followed patients with bipolar spectrum episodes for an extended period of time (ie, beyond the first year following TBI). Thus, uncertainty remains with regard to the prognosis and clinical course of persons with such episodes as well as the relationship of their symptoms to primary (idiopathic) bipolar disorder.

Risk Factors

The limited evidence and variable methods used to define and study bipolar and related mood disorders among persons with TBI preclude drawing definitive conclusions about risk factors for these conditions. In our study of early post-TBI mania, we observed no clear relationship between mixed episodes and TBI severity, posttraumatic epilepsy, post-TBI physical or cognitive impairments, level of social functioning, or the presence of family or personal history of psychiatric disorders.[75] Shukla and colleagues[76] also observed no relationship between posttraumatic mania and family history of bipolar disorder, but did note associations between post-TBI mania and injury severity (as estimated by duration of posttraumatic amnesia), as well as posttraumatic epilepsy. Complicating matters, the frequency of TBI may be elevated among unaffected family members of persons with bipolar disorder,[77] suggesting the possibility that heritable components of the bipolar phenotype (eg, increased novelty seeking, reduced harm avoidance, and impaired decision making) may increase the risk for TBI. Comorbid alcohol use disorders also affect the apparent, but not actual, risk for bipolar disorder among persons with TBI.[73]

Diagnostic Assessment

The DSM-V categorizes these disorders as bipolar and related disorders due to another medical condition (TBI) with (1) manic or hypomanic-like episode, (2) with manic features, and (3) with mixed features. Their diagnosis requires the unequivocal presence of a distinct period of abnormally and persistently elevated, expansive, or irritable mood lasting at least 4 days for hypomanic episodes or 1 week for manic episodes. Any other cognitive, vegetative, or behavioral disturbance counted toward that diagnosis must be either clearly related to the pervasive mood disturbance(s) or, if otherwise present, clearly exacerbated during the mood disturbance(s).

Overdiagnosis of mania and mixed states in this population is common in many clinical settings. This problem appears to derive most often from misattribution of

TBI-related disturbances in affect regulation (eg, frequent brief episodes of irritability or laughing), impulsive/disinhibited behaviors, alterations in sleep and appetitive behaviors, and cognitive disturbances to maniclike features despite the absence of the cardinal (mood) disturbance that the diagnosis requires. This distinction is not a matter of semantics: the treatment of paroxysmal disturbances of affect and disinhibited behaviors differ from those offered to persons with bipolar spectrum episodes. In particular, unopposed SSRIs are prescribed routinely and appropriately for the treatment of posttraumatic disturbances of affect and behavioral dyscontrol syndromes, a practice that is generally inadvisable among persons with secondary mania or mixed states.[78]

The methods used to diagnose manic or mixed episodes among persons with TBI are the same as those used to make primary (idiopathic) diagnoses of these types.[79] Using structured or semistructured psychiatric interviews to diagnose these conditions is encouraged, and the Young Mania Rating Scale[80] is useful as a measure of symptom severity and treatment response in this population.[81,82]

Differential Diagnosis

The differential diagnosis of mood disorders with manic, hypomanic, or mixed features among persons with TBI is broad and overlaps substantially with that of post-TBI depressive disorders. Several additional conditions merit consideration in this context, including emotional disturbances associated with delirium; mood disorders due to the effect of drugs, including intoxication and/or withdrawal states; posttraumatic epilepsy; and personality change due to TBI.

Transient euphoric and irritable symptoms may develop during the posttraumatic confusional state, during a post-TBI substance intoxication or withdrawal syndrome, or as a result of some medications, all of which preclude diagnosis of post-TBI mood disorder with manic, hypomanic, or mixed features. These symptoms rarely take on the appearance of true mania given their transience, lability, and co-occurrence with other symptoms of an acute confusional state. Such symptoms generally resolve in concert with the conditions in which they arise. When medication-induced maniclike or mixed-mood symptoms are suspected, medication taper and/or discontinuation are appropriate.

Posttraumatic epilepsy and its treatments are associated with the development of emotional disturbances, including maniclike symptoms and/or mixed mood states. Similarly, psychosis associated with epilepsy also may entail the concurrent development of emotional disturbances. Manic or mixed mood episodes that develop in this context may be temporally linked to seizures (or postictal psychosis) or may have a more prolonged course.

Finally, personality change due to TBI may include mood instability, disinhibited or impulsive behavior, and hyperactivity. These patients lack, however, the pervasive and sustained alteration of mood that characterizes manic or mixed syndromes.

Ancillary Studies

The evaluation of persons with TBI and suspected bipolar spectrum disorders follows the general principles and components of a complete psychiatric evaluation as outlined in the American Psychiatric Association's Practice Guideline for Psychiatric Evaluation of Adults.[83] Physical examination, including vital signs and a complete neurologic examination, is a requisite element of the initial evaluation.

As aforementioned, structural neuroimaging is a useful component of the evaluation of persons with TBI generally. However, more recent and refined neuroimaging techniques should be reserved for research at the present time. Video-EEG monitoring and

24-hour ambulatory recordings may be useful in the differential diagnosis of patients presenting with paroxysmal behavioral disturbances of unclear etiology or those that are associated with intra-episode or postepisode alterations of consciousness. This is particularly relevant to the evaluation of persons with TBI and mixed affective episodes in light of the possible associations between such disorders and posttraumatic epilepsy. Otherwise, neurophysiologic studies are not presently regarded as useful elements of the clinical evaluation in this context.

If the clinical history or examination suggest other endocrine or concurrent physical conditions, then performing problem-focused laboratory studies is appropriate.[47,84] In light of the relatively high frequency of neuroendocrine abnormalities in this population,[48] screening for thyroid dysfunction is encouraged as part of the initial evaluation. As with the evaluation of persons with depression, screening for human immunodeficiency virus infection as well as performing urine and/or serum toxicology screening for alcohol and other substances of abuse is encouraged.

Pharmacotherapy

The literature describing pharmacotherapy of bipolar spectrum disorders among persons with TBI is insufficient to permit the development of formal treatment guidelines.[61] Agents used to treat idiopathic manic and mixed mood states are used to treat bipolar spectrum disorders among persons with TBI. Clinicians are encouraged to refer to each medication's product information sheet as well as other reference materials for complete reviews of dosing, side effects, drug-drug interactions, treatment risks, and treatment contraindications before prescribing these or any other medications. The literature and common clinical experience suggests that most of these medications treat TBI-related manic and/or mixed mood states effectively. Their use in clinical practice therefore is informed by their side-effect profile.

Valproate may exacerbate cognitive impairments in some persons with TBI, but it appears less likely to do so than either carbamazepine or lithium.[85–87] Nonetheless, use of any of these agents necessitates careful and continuous assessment for the development of treatment-related motor (eg, tremor, ataxia, gait disturbances) and cognitive impairments, as well as other adverse side effects (eg, weight gain, gastrointestinal problems, hematologic abnormalities, hepatotoxicity, alopecia). Additionally, the risk of polycystic ovarian syndrome requires consideration of alternate treatments in women.

Given that lithium carbonate is used often as a first-line treatment among persons with idiopathic bipolar disorder, it merits special comment as a treatment of mixed states among persons with TBI. Intolerance of doses necessary to effect mood stabilization appears to be more common among persons with TBI than with primary mania or mixed mood episodes. This intolerance is often attributable to the adverse cognitive and motor effects of lithium carbonate, which appear more likely to produce nausea, tremor, ataxia, and lethargy in persons with neurologic disorders than in the general psychiatric population. Additionally, lithium carbonate lowers seizure threshold; in light of the risk for posttraumatic epilepsy as well as the potential comorbidity between posttraumatic epilepsy and mania, this effect is concerning with respect to lithium's use in this population. As such, partial response, relapse of symptoms, or need for a second mood-stabilizing medication are common limitations of the use of this agent among patients with TBI.

Several of the newer anticonvulsants (eg, lamotrigine, oxcarbazepine) and the atypical antipsychotics (eg, risperidone, olanzapine, ziprasidone, aripiprazole) may be useful in the treatment of posttraumatic manic, hypomanic and mixed states, but there are few published reports of their use. Clinicians interested in using these agents for this purpose are advised to undertake such treatments cautiously and with careful monitoring for adverse cognitive, motor, cardiac, and metabolic side effects.

In the absence of evidence demonstrating the superiority of one of these agents over the others, we generally recommend either valproate or quetiapine as first-line treatments, given their effectiveness for acute mania, rapid-cycling bipolar disorder, and antimanic prophylaxis, as well as their reasonable tolerability in persons with TBI. When these agents, alone or in combination, prove ineffective, then the use of one or more of the other agents may be required.

Psychotherapy

The TBI literature provides no clear guidance regarding the psychotherapeutic approach to persons with mania or mixed mood states after TBI. Education and supportive interventions regarding both TBI and also the mood disturbance with which the patient presents are reasonable and common-sense interventions. Additional psychotherapeutic interventions are modeled after those used in the management of persons with idiopathic bipolar disorders, as described in the American Psychiatric Association's practice guidelines for the treatment of patients with bipolar disorder.[84,88]

ECT and Brain-Stimulation Techniques

ECT appears to be effective for treatment-resistant or life-threatening manic or mixed mood episodes among persons with TBI. When ECT is selected as a treatment alternative, we recommend treatment with the lowest possible energy levels that will generate a seizure of adequate duration (greater than 20 seconds), using pulsatile currents, increased spacing of treatments (2 to 5 days between treatments), and fewer treatments in an entire course (ie, 4 to 6). In addition, if the patient also suffers from significant cognitive impairment due to TBI, unilateral ECT is the preferred technique. The role of other brain-stimulation techniques as treatment of these infrequent post-TBI disorders is uncertain at the present time, and the available evidence does not support their use.

SUMMARY AND FUTURE DIRECTIONS

Mood disorders are frequent psychiatric complications of TBI that overlap with prominent anxiety, substance misuse, impulsivity, and aggression. Furthermore, in a significant number of cases, they become chronic and resistant to treatment with the consequent deleterious impact on community reintegration and quality of life. Although the diagnosis of post-TBI mood disorders is still based on the DSM nomenclature, future nosology should incorporate the advances in neuroscience that are gradually allowing to parse the neural circuits whose disruption constitute the biologic substrate of the behavioral alterations associated with these conditions. Current therapeutic strategies are based on current standards of practice rather that empirically based controlled treatment trials. Randomized, double-blind, placebo-controlled trials to establish the most effective treatments for the variety of mood disorders associated with TBI are needed.

ACKNOWLEDGMENTS

The authors gratefully acknowledge the assistance of Ms Ashley Devereaux in the preparation of this article.

REFERENCES

1. Jorge RE, Robinson RG, Arndt SV, et al. Comparison between acute- and delayed-onset depression following traumatic brain injury. J Neuropsychiatry Clin Neurosci 1993;5(1):43–9.
2. Whelan-Goodinson R, Ponsford JL, Schonberger M, et al. Predictors of psychiatric disorders following traumatic brain injury. J Head Trauma Rehabil 2010; 25(5):320–9.
3. Seel RT, Macciocchi S, Kreutzer JS. Clinical considerations for the diagnosis of major depression after moderate to severe TBI. J Head Trauma Rehabil 2010; 25(2):99–112.
4. Kim E, Lauterbach EC, Reeve A, et al. Neuropsychiatric complications of traumatic brain injury: a critical review of the literature (a report by the ANPA Committee on Research). J Neuropsychiatry Clin Neurosci 2007;19(2): 106–27.
5. Koponen S, Taiminen T, Portin R, et al. Axis I and II psychiatric disorders after traumatic brain injury: a 30-year follow-up study. Am J Psychiatry 2002;159(8): 1315–21.
6. Hibbard MR, Uysal S, Kepler K, et al. Axis I psychopathology in individuals with traumatic brain injury. J Head Trauma Rehabil 1998;13(4):24–39.
7. Fedoroff JP, Starkstein SE, Forrester AW, et al. Depression in patients with acute traumatic brain injury. Am J Psychiatry 1992;149(7):918–23.
8. Jorge RE, Robinson RG, Moser D, et al. Major depression following traumatic brain injury. Arch Gen Psychiatry 2004;61(1):42–50.
9. Gould KR, Ponsford JL, Johnston L, et al. The nature, frequency and course of psychiatric disorders in the first year after traumatic brain injury: a prospective study. Psychol Med 2011;41(10):2099–109.
10. Tateno A, Jorge RE, Robinson RG. Clinical correlates of aggressive behavior after traumatic brain injury. J Neuropsychiatry Clin Neurosci 2003;15(2):155–60.
11. Bombardier CH, Fann JR, Temkin NR, et al. Rates of major depressive disorder and clinical outcomes following traumatic brain injury. JAMA 2010;303(19): 1938–45.
12. Hart T, Hoffman JM, Pretz C, et al. A longitudinal study of major and minor depression following traumatic brain injury. Arch Phys Med Rehabil 2012; 93(8):1343–9.
13. Deb S, Burns J. Neuropsychiatric consequences of traumatic brain injury: a comparison between two age groups. Brain Inj 2007;21(3):301–7.
14. Rapoport MJ, McCullagh S, Streiner D, et al. Age and major depression after mild traumatic brain injury. Am J Geriatr Psychiatry 2003;11(3):365–9.
15. Bay E, Sikorskii A, Saint-Arnault D. Sex differences in depressive symptoms and their correlates after mild-to-moderate traumatic brain injury. J Neurosci Nurs 2009;41(6):298–309 [quiz: 310–1].
16. Demakis GJ, Hammond FM, Knotts A. Prediction of depression and anxiety 1 year after moderate-severe traumatic brain injury. Appl Neuropsychol 2010; 17(3):183–9.
17. Koponen S, Taiminen T, Kairisto V, et al. APOE-epsilon4 predicts dementia but not other psychiatric disorders after traumatic brain injury. Neurology 2004; 63(4):749–50.
18. Caspi A, Sugden K, Moffitt TE, et al. Influence of life stress on depression: moderation by a polymorphism in the 5-HTT gene. Science 2003;301(5631): 386–9.

19. Arango V, Huang YY, Underwood MD, et al. Genetics of the serotonergic system in suicidal behavior. J Psychiatr Res 2003;37(5):375–86.
20. Binder EB, Salyakina D, Lichtner P, et al. Polymorphisms in FKBP5 are associated with increased recurrence of depressive episodes and rapid response to antidepressant treatment. Nat Genet 2004;36(12):1319–25.
21. Lotrich FE, Pollock BG. Meta-analysis of serotonin transporter polymorphisms and affective disorders. Psychiatr Genet 2004;14(3):121–9.
22. Patkar AA, Berrettini WH, Hoehe M, et al. Serotonin transporter polymorphisms and measures of impulsivity, aggression, and sensation seeking among African-American cocaine-dependent individuals. Psychiatry Res 2002;110(2):103–15.
23. Sen S, Villafuerte S, Nesse R, et al. Serotonin transporter and GABAA alpha 6 receptor variants are associated with neuroticism. Biol Psychiatry 2004;55(3):244–9.
24. Tunbridge E, Burnet PW, Sodhi MS, et al. Catechol-o-methyltransferase (COMT) and proline dehydrogenase (PRODH) mRNAs in the dorsolateral prefrontal cortex in schizophrenia, bipolar disorder, and major depression. Synapse 2004;51(2):112–8.
25. Zubenko GS, Maher B, Hughes HB 3rd, et al. Genome-wide linkage survey for genetic loci that influence the development of depressive disorders in families with recurrent, early-onset, major depression. Am J Med Genet B Neuropsychiatr Genet 2003;123(1):1–18.
26. Lasky-Su JA, Faraone SV, Glatt SJ, et al. Meta-analysis of the association between two polymorphisms in the serotonin transporter gene and affective disorders. Am J Med Genet B Neuropsychiatr Genet 2005;133(1):110–5.
27. Sun HS, Tsai HW, Ko HC, et al. Association of tryptophan hydroxylase gene polymorphism with depression, anxiety and comorbid depression and anxiety in a population-based sample of postpartum Taiwanese women. Genes Brain Behav 2004;3(6):328–36.
28. Smith GS, Lotrich FE, Malhotra AK, et al. Effects of serotonin transporter promoter polymorphisms on serotonin function. Neuropsychopharmacology 2004;29(12):2226–34.
29. McAllister TW, Flashman LA, Harker Rhodes C, et al. Single nucleotide polymorphisms in ANKK1 and the dopamine D2 receptor gene affect cognitive outcome shortly after traumatic brain injury: a replication and extension study. Brain Inj 2008;22(9):705–14.
30. Lipsky RH, Sparling MB, Ryan LM, et al. Association of COMT Val158Met genotype with executive functioning following traumatic brain injury. J Neuropsychiatry Clin Neurosci 2005;17(4):465–71.
31. Chan F, Lanctot KL, Feinstein A, et al. The serotonin transporter polymorphisms and major depression following traumatic brain injury. Brain Inj 2008;22(6):471–9.
32. Lanctot KL, Rapoport MJ, Chan F, et al. Genetic predictors of response to treatment with citalopram in depression secondary to traumatic brain injury. Brain Inj 2010;24(7–8):959–69.
33. Heim C, Newport DJ, Bonsall R, et al. Altered pituitary-adrenal axis responses to provocative challenge tests in adult survivors of childhood abuse. Am J Psychiatry 2001;158(4):575–81.
34. Heim C, Newport DJ, Heit S, et al. Pituitary-adrenal and autonomic responses to stress in women after sexual and physical abuse in childhood. JAMA 2000;284(5):592–7.

35. Jorge RE, Robinson RG, Arndt SV, et al. Depression following traumatic brain injury: a 1 year longitudinal study. J Affect Disord 1993;27(4):233–43.
36. Fann JR, Burington B, Leonetti A, et al. Psychiatric illness following traumatic brain injury in an adult health maintenance organization population. Arch Gen Psychiatry 2004;61(1):53–61.
37. Jorge RE, Starkstein SE, Arndt S, et al. Alcohol misuse and mood disorders following traumatic brain injury. Arch Gen Psychiatry 2005;62(7):742–9.
38. Starkstein SE, Lischinsky A. The phenomenology of depression after brain injury. NeuroRehabilitation 2002;17(2):105–13.
39. Fann JR, Bombardier CH, Dikmen S, et al. Validity of the Patient Health Questionnaire-9 in assessing depression following traumatic brain injury. J Head Trauma Rehabil 2005;20(6):501–11.
40. Green A, Felmingham K, Baguley IJ, et al. The clinical utility of the Beck Depression Inventory after traumatic brain injury. Brain Inj 2001;15(12):1021–8.
41. Seel RT, Kreutzer JS. Depression assessment after traumatic brain injury: an empirically based classification method. Arch Phys Med Rehabil 2003;84(11):1621–8.
42. Whelan-Goodinson R, Ponsford J, Johnston L, et al. Psychiatric disorders following traumatic brain injury: their nature and frequency. J Head Trauma Rehabil 2009;24(5):324–32.
43. Kant R, Duffy JD, Pivovarnik A. Prevalence of apathy following head injury. Brain Inj 1998;12(1):87–92.
44. Marin RS, Fogel BS, Hawkins J, et al. Apathy: a treatable syndrome. J Neuropsychiatry Clin Neurosci 1995;7(1):23–30.
45. Larson MJ, Kaufman DA, Kellison IL, et al. Double jeopardy! The additive consequences of negative affect on performance-monitoring decrements following traumatic brain injury. Neuropsychology 2009;23(4):433–44.
46. Reza MF, Ikoma K, Ito T, et al. N200 latency and P300 amplitude in depressed mood post-traumatic brain injury patients. Neuropsychol Rehabil 2007;17(6):723–34.
47. American Psychiatric Association. Treatment of patients with major depressive disorder, in APA practice guidelines, major depressive disorder. American Psychiatric Association; 2010. Available at: http://www.psych.org/practice/clinical-practice-guidelines.
48. Rothman MS, Arciniegas DB, Filley CM, et al. The neuroendocrine effects of traumatic brain injury. J Neuropsychiatry Clin Neurosci 2007;19(4):363–72.
49. Bell KR, Hoffman JM, Temkin NR, et al. The effect of telephone counselling on reducing post-traumatic symptoms after mild traumatic brain injury: a randomised trial. J Neurol Neurosurg Psychiatr 2008;79(11):1275–81.
50. Snell DL, Surgenor LJ, Hay-Smith EJ, et al. A systematic review of psychological treatments for mild traumatic brain injury: an update on the evidence. J Clin Exp Neuropsychol 2009;31(1):20–38.
51. Anson K, Ponsford J. Evaluation of a coping skills group following traumatic brain injury. Brain Inj 2006;20(2):167–78.
52. Anson K, Ponsford J. Who benefits? Outcome following a coping skills group intervention for traumatically brain injured individuals. Brain Inj 2006;20(1):1–13.
53. Hegel MT, Ferguson RJ. Differential reinforcement of other behavior (DRO) to reduce aggressive behavior following traumatic brain injury. Behav Modif 2000;24(1):94–101.

54. Delmonico RL, Hanley-Peterson P, Englander J. Group psychotherapy for persons with traumatic brain injury: management of frustration and substance abuse. J Head Trauma Rehabil 1998;13(6):10–22.
55. Bell KR, Hoffman JM, Doctor JN, et al. Development of a telephone follow-up program for individuals following traumatic brain injury. J Head Trauma Rehabil 2004;19(6):502–12.
56. Kurowski BG, Wade SL, Kirkwood MW, et al. Online problem-solving therapy for executive dysfunction after child traumatic brain injury. Pediatrics 2013;132(1): e158–66.
57. Hibbard MR, Cantor J, Charatz H, et al. Peer support in the community: initial findings of a mentoring program for individuals with traumatic brain injury and their families. J Head Trauma Rehabil 2002;17(2):112–31.
58. Groom KN, Shaw TG, O'Connor ME, et al. Neurobehavioral symptoms and family functioning in traumatically brain-injured adults. Arch Clin Neuropsychol 1998;13(8):695–711.
59. Harris JK, Godfrey HP, Partridge FM, et al. Caregiver depression following traumatic brain injury (TBI): a consequence of adverse effects on family members? Brain Inj 2001;15(3):223–38.
60. Leach LR, Frank RG, Bouman DE, et al. Family functioning, social support and depression after traumatic brain injury. Brain Inj 1994;8(7):599–606.
61. Warden DL, Gordon B, McAllister TW, et al. Guidelines for the pharmacologic treatment of neurobehavioral sequelae of traumatic brain injury. J Neurotrauma 2006;23(10):1468–501.
62. Kant R, Smith-Seemiller L, Zeiler D. Treatment of aggression and irritability after head injury. Brain Inj 1998;12(8):661–6.
63. Fann JR, Uomoto JM, Katon WJ. Sertraline in the treatment of major depression following mild traumatic brain injury. J Neuropsychiatry Clin Neurosci 2000; 12(2):226–32.
64. Fann JR, Uomoto JM, Katon WJ. Cognitive improvement with treatment of depression following mild traumatic brain injury. Psychosomatics 2001;42(1):48–54.
65. Schmitt JA, Kruizinga MJ, Riedel WJ. Non-serotonergic pharmacological profiles and associated cognitive effects of serotonin reuptake inhibitors. J Psychopharmacol 2001;15(3):173–9.
66. Lee H, Kim SW, Kim JM, et al. Comparing effects of methylphenidate, sertraline and placebo on neuropsychiatric sequelae in patients with traumatic brain injury. Hum Psychopharmacol 2005;20(2):97–104.
67. Gualtieri CT, Evans RW. Stimulant treatment for the neurobehavioural sequelae of traumatic brain injury. Brain Inj 1988;2(4):273–90.
68. Alper K, Schwartz KA, Kolts RL, et al. Seizure incidence in psychopharmacological clinical trials: an analysis of Food and Drug Administration (FDA) summary basis of approval reports. Biol Psychiatry 2007;62(4):345–54.
69. Kraus MF, Maki PM. Effect of amantadine hydrochloride on symptoms of frontal lobe dysfunction in brain injury: case studies and review. J Neuropsychiatry Clin Neurosci 1997;9(2):222–30.
70. Meythaler JM, Brunner RC, Johnson A, et al. Amantadine to improve neurorecovery in traumatic brain injury-associated diffuse axonal injury: a pilot double-blind randomized trial. J Head Trauma Rehabil 2002;17(4):300–13.
71. Giacino JT, Whyte J, Bagiella E, et al. Placebo-controlled trial of amantadine for severe traumatic brain injury. N Engl J Med 2012;366(9):819–26.
72. Demirtas-Tatlidede A, Vahabzadeh-Hagh AM, Bernabeu M, et al. Noninvasive brain stimulation in traumatic brain injury. J Head Trauma Rehabil 2012;27(4):274–92.

73. Silver JM, Kramer R, Greenwald S, et al. The association between head injuries and psychiatric disorders: findings from the New Haven NIMH Epidemiologic Catchment Area Study. Brain Inj 2001;15(11):935–45.

74. van Reekum R, Cohen T, Wong J. Can traumatic brain injury cause psychiatric disorders? J Neuropsychiatry Clin Neurosci 2000;12(3):316–27.

75. Jorge RE, Robinson RG, Starkstein SE, et al. Secondary mania following traumatic brain injury. Am J Psychiatry 1993;150(6):916–21.

76. Shukla S, Cook BL, Mukherjee S, et al. Mania following head trauma. Am J Psychiatry 1987;144(1):93–6.

77. Malaspina D, Goetz RR, Friedman JH, et al. Traumatic brain injury and schizophrenia in members of schizophrenia and bipolar disorder pedigrees. Am J Psychiatry 2001;158(3):440–6.

78. Dealberto MJ, Marino J, Bourgon L. Homicidal ideation with intent during a manic episode triggered by antidepressant medication in a man with brain injury. Bipolar Disord 2008;10(1):111–3.

79. Jorge R, Robinson RG. Mood disorders following traumatic brain injury. Int Rev Psychiatry 2003;15(4):317–27.

80. Young RC, Biggs JT, Ziegler VE, et al. A rating scale for mania: reliability, validity and sensitivity. Br J Psychiatry 1978;133:429–35.

81. Oster TJ, Anderson CA, Filley CM, et al. Quetiapine for mania due to traumatic brain injury. CNS Spectr 2007;12(10):764–9.

82. Daniels JP, Felde A. Quetiapine treatment for mania secondary to brain injury in 2 patients. J Clin Psychiatry 2008;69(3):497–8.

83. American Psychiatric Association. Practice guideline for psychiatric evaluation of adults. Am J Psychiatry 1995;152(Suppl 11):63–80.

84. Hirschfeld RM. Guideline watch: practice guideline for the treatment of patients with bipolar disorder. APA Practice Guidelines. 2002. http://dx.doi.org/10.1176/appi.books.9780890423363.148430.

85. Dikmen SS, Machamer JE, Winn HR, et al. Neuropsychological effects of valproate in traumatic brain injury: a randomized trial. Neurology 2000;54(4):895–902.

86. Massagli TL. Neurobehavioral effects of phenytoin, carbamazepine, and valproic acid: implications for use in traumatic brain injury. Arch Phys Med Rehabil 1991;72(3):219–26.

87. Hornstein A, Seliger G. Cognitive side effects of lithium in closed head injury. J Neuropsychiatry Clin Neurosci 1989;1(4):446–7.

88. American Psychiatric Association. Practice guideline for the treatment of patients with bipolar disorder (revision). Am J Psychiatry 2002;159(Suppl 4):1–50.

Emotional and Behavioral Dyscontrol After Traumatic Brain Injury

David B. Arciniegas, MD[a,b,c,*], Hal S. Wortzel, MD[a,c,d]

KEYWORDS

- Pathological laughing and crying • Affective lability • Irritability • Management
- Aggression • Traumatic brain injury • Assessment • Disinhibition

KEY POINTS

- Emotional dyscontrol is a common consequence of traumatic brain injury (TBI) and includes pathologic laughing and crying (also known as *pseudobulbar affect* or *emotional incontinence*), affective lability, and irritability. These problems are common in the early period following mild TBI, after which they resolve in most people. Emotional dyscontrol is a common acute and chronic problem among persons with moderate or severe TBI.
- Among the most challenging forms of posttraumatic behavioral dyscontrol are disinhibition and aggression. These problems tend to be more common, chronic, disruptive, and challenging to manage among persons with moderate and severe TBI.
- Emotional and behavioral dyscontrol frequently co-occur with other posttraumatic neuropsychiatric disturbances, the treatment of which may concurrently reduce the frequency and severity of dyscontrol symptoms.
- When emotional and/or behavioral dyscontrol require symptom-specific treatments, a combination of nonpharmacologic (ie, psychological, behavioral, environmental) and pharmacologic approaches is usually required. Properly administered, these interventions may provide persons with TBI and their families with substantial relief from these problems and their effects on daily functioning and quality of life.

Support for this work was provided by National Institute on Disability and Rehabilitation Research (NIDRR) grants H133A120020 and H133A130047 (D.B. Arciniegas) and the Veterans Health Administration's VISN-19 MIRECC (H.S. Wortzel). The content of this article is the sole responsibility of the authors and does not necessarily represent the official views of the Department of Veterans Affairs or NIDRR.
[a] Beth K. and Stuart C. Yudofsky Division of Neuropsychiatry, Menninger Department of Psychiatry and Behavioral Sciences, Baylor College of Medicine, Houston, TX, USA; [b] Brain Injury Research Center, TIRR Memorial Hermann, Houston, TX, USA; [c] Neuropsychiatry Service, Department of Psychiatry, University of Colorado School of Medicine, Aurora, CO, USA; [d] VISN 19 MIRECC, Denver Veterans Medical Center, Denver, CO, USA
* Corresponding author. TIRR Memorial Hermann Research Center, 1333 Moursund Street, Room 202, Houston, TX 77030.
E-mail address: david.arciniegas@bcm.edu

Acronyms	
CDEs	Common data elements
CNS-LS	Center for Neurologic Study-Lability Scale
DSM-5	Diagnostic and Statistical Manual of Mental Disorders, Fifth Edition
ICD-9-CM	International Classification of Diseases, 9th Edition, Clinical Modification
NINDS	National Institute of Neurological Disorders and Stroke
NPI	Neuropsychiatric Inventory
NPI-C	Neuropsychiatric Inventory-Clinician
NPI-Q	Neuropsychiatric Inventory-Questionnaire
PAI	Personality Assessment Inventory
PLACS	Pathological Laughter and Crying Scale
PLC	Pathological laughing and crying
SSRI	Selective serotonin reuptake inhibitor
TBI	Traumatic brain injury

Traumatic brain injury (TBI) is associated with a broad range of emotional and behavioral disturbances during both the early and late postinjury periods.[1,2] Neuropsychiatric disturbances of these types include depression, secondary mania, anxiety, affective lability, irritability, disinhibition, restlessness and agitation, aggression, and apathy, among others. Emotional dyscontrol (which, for the purposes of this article, refers to pathologic laughing and crying, affective lability, and irritability) as well as behavioral dyscontrol (here denoting disinhibition and aggression) are challenging for persons with TBI, their families and caregivers, and health care professionals serving to understand and address these conditions.[3–9]

In the early period following TBI, emotional and behavioral disturbances may be symptoms of posttraumatic encephalopathy (reflecting neurotrauma-induced diffuse brain dysfunction)[10–16] and/or manifestations of focal injuries to brain systems subserving emotional regulation and comportment.[10–16] These disturbances are especially common among individuals whose initial injuries are severe enough to require hospitalization and inpatient rehabilitation.[10,11,15,16] In this population, emotional and behavioral disturbances tend to improve with time but may become chronic and functionally limiting problems for some persons with TBI.[3–5,17,18]

Emotional and behavioral dyscontrol (eg, affective lability, irritability, restlessness, agitation) may also occur in the early period following mild TBI.[19] When such problems develop in this population, they typically are most severe in the immediate postinjury period[20] and may reflect the presence of focal lesions or comorbidities requiring immediate medical evaluation.[19,21] As with other symptoms of concussion, these problems are usually transient and, in most persons with mild TBI, typically resolve in the first several postinjury weeks.[20,22]

In some cases, emotional and behavioral dyscontrol are manifestations of another psychiatric condition (eg, major depressive episode, manic, hypomanic, or mixed episode, posttraumatic stress disorder, anxiety disorders, substance use disorders, psychotic disorders),[7,23–32] including recurrence or exacerbation of preinjury psychiatric disorders.[20,33] Physical problems, especially pain,[30,31,34,35] and medications with adverse behavioral effects[35,36] also may contribute to emotional and behavioral dyscontrol among persons with TBI.

Although treating comorbid psychiatric, substance use, physical, and psychosocial problems may reduce or eliminate emotional and behavioral dyscontrol, these will remain distressing and functionally limiting symptoms for some persons with TBI.[3–7,18] In such circumstances, emotional and behavioral dyscontrol become distinct targets of pharmacologic and other rehabilitative treatments. Unfortunately, and in contrast to pharmacotherapies[37–41] and rehabilitation[42–46] for persons with cognitive deficits after TBI, the evidence bases for treatments of posttraumatic emotional and behavioral dyscontrol are underdeveloped.[37,40,41,47]

In the service of providing clinicians with practical guidance on the evaluation and management of these problems, this article provides working definitions of these categories of neuropsychiatric disturbance. Methods of assessing emotional and behavioral dyscontrol are described briefly, and the importance of considering the differential diagnoses for these clinical phenomena is highlighted. Pharmacologic and nonpharmacologic treatments for emotional and behavioral dyscontrol, derived from a synthesis of the literature and the experience of the authors, then are outlined.

EMOTIONAL DYSCONTROL

Emotional dyscontrol denotes a tendency to display unpredictable and rapidly changing emotions. It encompasses several disorders of affect, including pathologic laughing and crying (PLC), affective lability, and irritability. These disorders are not specific to TBI[48,49] but occur among persons with TBI with sufficient frequency and clinical import to require treatment.[47,50–58]

These conditions may be assigned *Diagnostic and Statistical Manual of Mental Disorders, Fifth Edition (DSM-5)*[59] code 310.1, personality change due to another medical condition, labile type. Alternatively, conditions in the category of emotional dyscontrol may be assigned *International Classification of Diseases, Ninth Revision, Clinical Modification (ICD-9-CM)*[60] diagnosis code 301.3, which corresponds to the descriptor synonyms *pathologic emotionality* or *emotional instability, excessive*.

Pathological Laughing and Crying

The prototypical form of emotional dyscontrol is PLC, also known as *pseudobulbar affect* or *emotional incontinence*.[48,61–63] PLC is a disorder of affect associated with neurologic conditions, such as TBI, and involves a severe disturbance in moment-to-moment emotional experience and expression rather than the sustained, excessive, and pervasive disturbances characteristic of mood disorders (eg, depression, dysthymia, secondary mania).[48,49,59] This condition is defined by the occurrence of brief, stereotyped, intense, uncontrollable episodes of laughing and/or crying (ie, emotional expression) that are triggered by sentimentally trivial or neutral stimuli and that do not bear a predictable relationship to the emotional feeling state during or between the moments of abnormal emotional expression. These episodes must produce subjective distress or interfere with everyday function to merit diagnosis and treatment.[49,53]

The incidence and prevalence of PLC among persons with TBI are not well established. The reported frequency of PLC during the first year after injury is 5% to 11%.[51,57] Common clinical experience suggests that the frequency of PLC may be less than these reported frequencies and tends to decline further in the late postinjury period. The prevalence of PLC in the late period following TBI is not known, however, and there are some individuals, especially those with relatively severe TBI involving the dorsolateral and anterior frontal cortices, internal capsule, and/or pontocerebellar structures,[63,64] for whom this becomes a chronic condition.

PLC may co-occur with mood disorders (especially depression), anxiety disorders, and behavioral dyscontrol (ie, aggression) among persons with TBI.[51] Structured interview using the Pathologic Laughter and Crying Scale (PLACS)[65] facilitates the identification of episodes of emotional dyscontrol characteristic of PLC from emotional expressions and experiences that are more consistent with depression or mixed depression-anxiety. PLC must also be distinguished from a form of normal emotionalism known as *essential crying*[66] and from personality disorders (eg, borderline and/or histrionic personality disorders). Essential crying is a relatively uncommon, lifelong, and (probably) hereditary propensity for crying in response to stimuli of modest sentimental value that lies at the border between normal affective variability and abnormal emotional expression (ie, affective lability). Essential crying is not usually experienced as distressing or functionally limiting and therefore does not require treatment. Personality disorder–related disturbances of affect are distinguished from PLC by their nonstereotyped and less discretely paroxysmal character, predictable correspondence between in-the-moment emotional expression and experience, and tendency to develop in relation to personally or interpersonally relevant stimuli.

PLC also may co-occur with epilepsy among persons with TBI[52] and must be distinguished from ictal laughing (gelastic seizure) and ictal crying (dacrystic or quiritarian seizure). These seizures are partial-onset seizures in which the seizure itself produces laughing or crying. They involve ictal alteration of consciousness and at least a brief period of postictal confusion, which serve to distinguish them phenomenologically from PLC. However, video-electroencephalogram monitoring of these events may be required to clearly differentiate between these conditions.

Clinical interview of the person with TBI and a knowledgeable informant coupled with serial observations of the patient are usually sufficient to establish a diagnosis of PLC. Among patients with relatively modest cognitive deficits and preserved self-awareness, administration of the PLACS[65] is useful for diagnosing this condition, characterizing its severity, and monitoring response to treatment. The Center for Neurologic Study-Lability Scale (CNS-LS)[67] is a self-report measure that also may be useful for this purpose, although the items on this measure are explicitly directed at identifying affective lability rather than PLC. It therefore may be useful to regard the CNS-LS as a self-report screening measure for symptoms suggestive of PLC and to follow up positive screens on this measure with an interview using the PLACS.

Among patients with more severe cognitive and/or self-awareness deficits, structured interview of a knowledgeable informant using the Neuropsychiatric Inventory (NPI)[68–71] is a useful method of screening for symptoms of PLC. When responses to the dysphoria and/or elation subscales of the NPI suggest the possibility of PLC, using the PLACS as a guide to the continued interview of the informant usefully clarifies whether those symptoms are consistent with PLC.

When the diagnosis of PLC is made, explaining the diagnosis and providing support to the affected person and his or her family is important and usually helpful. The first-line treatment of PLC, however, is pharmacotherapy. The literature regarding this condition consistently demonstrates that serotonergically and/or noradrenergically active antidepressants are effective treatments of PLC involving episodes of crying, laughing, or both.[49] In light of their ease of use and relatively benign side-effect profiles at the relatively low doses required to affect symptomatic improvement, the selective serotonin reuptake inhibitors (SSRIs) are the first-line treatments for PLC among persons with TBI.[55] Sertraline, citalopram, and escitalopram are favored for this purpose in light of their relatively short half-lives, limited drug-drug and CYP450 interactions, and generally favorable side-effect profiles.[49]

If these agents are not effective, then augmentation with (or switching to) another medication may be required. Among those used for these purposes in persons with TBI are methylphenidate (especially with comorbid inattention and/or slow processing speed)[72]; lamotrigine (especially with comorbid epilepsy)[52]; levodopa or amantadine[73]; and anticonvulsants, such as valproate or carbamazepine (especially with comorbid irritability/anger, aggressive, and/or self-destructive behaviors).[50,74]

Dextromethorphan-quinidine is also an option for the treatment of PLC due to TBI.[49] However, there are no published data regarding this agent's safety and tolerability (especially with regard to cognitive effects) among persons with TBI, and its quinidine component entails a substantial risk of problematic drug-drug interactions. Pending publication of data that inform on these concerns, prudence dictates that this compound be used to treat posttraumatic PLC only when other agents are ineffective or intolerable.

Affective Lability

Affective lability (also known as *emotional lability*) refers to a tendency to be easily overcome with intense emotions in response to personally or socially meaningful stimuli or events that ordinarily would induce more modest emotional responses.[48,75–77] Affective lability manifests as brief, nonstereotyped episodes of congruent emotional expression and experience that are not discretely paroxysmal, of variable intensity, and partially amenable to voluntary control or interruption by external events (ie, distractors). Affective lability characteristically involves crying or laughing but may also entail anxiety and/or irritability.[78] Although episodes of affective lability are not stereotyped to the same degree as those of PLC, they involve emotional expressions and experiences that are more stereotyped than normal.[79] Similar to PLC, affective lability does not necessarily reflect the presence of a mood disorder and does not produce a persistent change in mood.

The reported prevalence of affective lability among persons with TBI is highly variable, at least in part reflecting differences in case definitions, assessment methods, injury severity, time since injury, and ascertainment biases. Among persons with mild TBI, affective lability may be as high as 28% in the first week to three months after injury.[80] However, most concussion symptom inventories do not query about affective lability specifically and instead capture symptoms like irritability, nervousness, depression, and anxiety,[81–84] leaving uncertain the actual frequency of this problem in the early and late postconcussive periods. Among persons with severe TBI, estimates of the prevalence of affectively lability (referred to as *mood swings* or *lability of mood* in some reports) range from 33% to 46%[15,85] in the early postinjury period to 14% to 62% in the late postinjury period.[85–87]

The evaluation of affective lability among individuals capable of providing reliable self-report is guided usefully by the affective lability scale[88] or the CNS-LS.[67] The affective lability scale is a lengthier instrument than the CNS-LS and provides for a more detailed characterization of this problem. The CNS-LS is shorter and may be the more practical of these measures to use in daily practice. Among persons with severe cognitive impairments or self-awareness deficits, the NPI[68–71] provides a framework for an informant-based interview that facilitates identification and serial evaluation of affective lability via items in the dysphoria, elation, and irritability/lability subscales. The NPI-Clinician version (NPI-C)[71] may be particularly useful for this purpose in light of its integrated informant-based and clinician-observed approaches to neuropsychiatric symptom identification and characterization.

Affective lability is not specific to TBI or to traditionally defined neurologic disorders and instead is observed in association with a broad range of psychiatric and medical problems.[50] Affective lability also occurs during depressive and dysthymic episodes,[89] the euthymic period of bipolar disorder,[77,90–92] substance use disorders,[78] and among individuals with idiopathic personality disorders.[88,89,92–95] The evaluation of affective lability among persons with TBI therefore requires consideration of the broad differential diagnosis for this problem and especially the possibility of a concurrent mood and/or personality disorder.

The treatment of affective lability employs nonpharmacologic and pharmacologic approaches. Counseling and education focused on improving self-efficacy and self-regulation are commonly provided and reasonable initial interventions.[96,97] Structured rehabilitation interventions focused on concurrently improving emotional regulation and cognitive performance are beneficial,[98–101] and their provisional use (and further study) in patients with comorbid posttraumatic cognitive impairments and emotional dyscontrol, including affective lability, is suggested.

Pharmacotherapies of posttraumatic affective lability are similar to those used to treat posttraumatic PLC. Serotonergically active antidepressants are first-line interventions for this problem and are usually effective and tolerated well.[48] Sertraline, citalopram, and escitalopram are favored for this purpose in light of their relatively short half-lives, limited drug-drug and CYP-450 interactions, and generally favorable side-effect profiles.[49] If SSRIs are partially effective or ineffective, then treatment with another medication may be necessary. The potential options include methylphenidate (especially for patients with comorbid inattention and/or slow processing speed); amantadine (especially with comorbid irritability and/or aggression); anticonvulsants, such as valproate or carbamazepine (especially with comorbid irritability/anger, aggressive, and/or self-destructive behaviors); or lamotrigine (especially with comorbid epilepsy). The preliminary evidence suggests that valproate or carbamazepine may also be useful for the treatment of co-occurring affective lability (especially anxious-irritable type) and alcohol dependence after TBI.[78] There are no data demonstrating the benefits of dextromethorphan-quinidine on posttraumatic affective lability, and its use for this purpose is not recommended.

Irritability

Irritability and associated symptoms (eg, annoyance, impatience, anger, loss of temper) are common in the general population[102] and tend to increase in frequency and/or severity after mild, moderate, or severe TBI.[103–109] Alderman (2003)[110] notes that the term *irritable* refers both to an internal experience (ie, becoming annoyed easily) as well as overt expressions reflecting that experience (ie, showing anger). Eames (2001)[111] suggested that posttraumatic irritability in the early postinjury period is characterized by snappiness, with irritability arising in response to nearly any stressor or frustration, and that this problem tends to resolve over time. By contrast, irritability in the late postinjury period is characterized by recurrent, transient, ego-dystonic outbursts that are triggered by unpredictable and trivial stimuli and represent a change from preinjury affective responding (ie, such responses are "out of character").[111]

Conceptually, posttraumatic irritability is more consistent with a disorder of affect than a mood disorder.[48,49,59] Posttraumatic irritability reflects disturbances of moment-to-moment emotion (ie, the "emotional weather" or affect) rather than a persistent change in baseline emotion (ie, the "emotional climate" or mood). Although patients with posttraumatic irritability are prone to experience and express transient irritation, impatience, anger, and/or loss of temper in response to the events of daily life, their emotional state between episodes of irritation is often relatively neutral (ie, they do not experience sustained, excessive, and context-independent irritability or anger).

In one of the earliest reports describing posttraumatic irritability, McKinlay and colleagues[85] (1981) identified irritability as one of several forms of loss of emotional control occurring in persons with moderate and severe TBI (ie, at least two days of posttraumatic amnesia). In their sample of 55 subjects, 63%, 69%, and 71% demonstrated irritability at 3, 6, and 12 months, respectively. The majority of individuals with posttraumatic irritability also demonstrated bad temper (ie, anger outbursts), impatience, tension and anxiety, affective lability, and depressive-type symptoms. Deb and colleagues[87] (1999) interviewed 196 individuals approximately one year after hospitalization-requiring TBI of at least complicated mild severity and observed irritability in 35%. This symptom frequently co-occurred with other symptoms of emotional and behavioral dyscontrol, including impatience, mood swings (ie, affective lability), and verbal outbursts, similar to the observations of McKinlay and colleagues[85] (1981) and others.[4,82,83,103,106,107] Among persons with mild TBI, irritability is a common postconcussive symptom in the early postinjury period.[4,82,83,106,107] In most individuals with such injuries, this symptom improves over time such that it occurs at a frequency comparable to that among persons without TBI.[20,103,107]

As a result of the commonplace occurrence of irritability and associated symptoms in the general population,[102] the presence of these symptoms after TBI cannot be unequivocally attributed to TBI. Preinjury emotionality, comorbid psychiatric disorders (especially dysphoric depression, irritable mania/hypomania, mixed mood episode, anxiety disorders, posttraumatic stress disorder), substance use, pain, and medications may contribute to or explain irritability among persons with TBI.[7,23–32,112] When present, each of these problems may be a more appropriate first target of treatment than irritability itself, and their effective treatment may obviate treatments targeting irritability specifically.[25] Evaluation of irritability and associated symptoms among patients with histories of TBI therefore needs to include consideration of contributing or explanatory preinjury and postinjury neuropsychiatric comorbidities and/or contemporaneous psychosocial stressors.

The evaluation of people with posttraumatic irritability and associated symptoms also requires consideration of potential influence of co-occurring cognitive and self-awareness deficits.[103,109,113,114] Yang and colleagues[103,113] (2012, 2013) consistently observed greater self-reported irritability among persons with mild TBI than among those with moderate to severe TBI, and the reported frequencies of irritability among persons with moderate to severe TBI did not differ from those of healthy comparators.[103] However, the frequency of caregiver-reported irritability among persons with moderate to severe TBI is comparable with that self-reported by those with mild TBI, both of which were higher than the frequency reported by persons without TBI.[103,113] Deficits in self-awareness among persons with moderate to severe TBI were suggested as the probable cause of this discrepancy in self-reported versus informant-reported posttraumatic irritability. These observations suggest that different methods of neuropsychiatric evaluation may be required to identify, characterize, and monitor changes in posttraumatic irritability in persons with mild versus moderate-to-severe TBI.

Among patients with preserved self-awareness after TBI, self-report measures like the Neurobehavioral Symptom Inventory,[82,83] the Irritability Questionnaire,[115] or the National Taiwan University Irritability Scale[116] may be useful assessments of posttraumatic irritability. The Neurobehavioral Symptom Inventory is a multi-symptom assessment scale that is included in the National Institute of Neurological Disorders and Stroke (NINDS) Common Data Elements (CDEs) for TBI (version 2.01).[117] This scale includes an irritability item and a frustration item, each of which is self-rated on a 5-point Likert scale. This measure is useful for identifying irritability and frustration but is relatively limited with regard to its characterization of these problems. It therefore may be most useful as a screening measure for irritability and, when this problem is identified, supplemented with a symptom-specific measure (eg, the Irritability Questionnaire or National Taiwan University Irritability Scale).

Among patients with limited self-awareness after TBI, informant-based assessment of irritability is recommended. The NPI appears to provide useful informant-based ratings of functionally important levels of irritability among persons with TBI.[6,7,118,119] Although the NPI has not yet been adopted into the NINDS CDEs for TBI specifically,[117] the questionnaire (NPI-Q)[70] version of this measure is incorporated into the August 2013 revisions to the NINDS General CDEs (ie, those intended for use in all neurologic conditions). The use of the NPI to identify, characterize, and monitor treatment-related changes in posttraumatic irritability therefore is recommended.

Options for treating posttraumatic irritability and associated symptoms include pharmacotherapy and psychotherapy. Nonpharmacologic interventions are appropriately regarded as first-line for this purpose, especially among patients with mild or moderate irritability symptoms and relatively preserved cognition. Useful approaches include counseling and psychotherapy[120] as well as a manualized form of anger self-management training developed specifically for persons with TBI.[121] Group cognitive behavioral therapy, modified to accommodate posttraumatic cognitive impairments, also reduces the frequency of experienced and expressed anger among persons with severe TBI.[122] Structured rehabilitation interventions that focus concurrently on improving emotional self-regulation and functional cognitive performance are beneficial,[98–101] and their application to the treatment of patients with comorbid posttraumatic irritability and cognitive impairments is encouraged.

Severe irritability and associated symptoms may require adjunctive pharmacotherapy. When an individual with posttraumatic irritability is unable to engage effectively in symptom-targeted nonpharmacologic treatments, pharmacotherapy may be the principal method of treatment. When effective, it also may facilitate participation in counseling, psychotherapy, or behavioral therapies. Published case reports or case series describe sertraline,[123] valproate,[124] methylphenidate,[72] carbamazepine,[125] quetiapine,[126] aripiprazole,[127] buspirone,[128] propranolol,[129] and homeopathic medications[130] as beneficial treatments for posttraumatic irritability. A recently published parallel-group, randomized, double-blind, placebo-controlled trial of amantadine for chronic posttraumatic irritability and aggression in 76 individuals more than 6 months post injury demonstrated significant reductions in irritability as assessed by the NPI (81% of those receiving this agent versus 44% on placebo). This treatment was tolerated well, and adverse effect types and frequencies did not differ from placebo; however, one participant required amantadine discontinuation because of seizure. This study suggests a potentially important role for amantadine in the treatment of chronic posttraumatic irritability, and publication of results of a multicenter randomized controlled trial that clarify the role of amantadine in the treatment of this condition is anticipated in the near future (see http://clinicaltrials.gov/show/NCT00779324).

BEHAVIORAL DYSCONTROL

Behavioral dyscontrol denotes a tendency to act impulsively in response to internal or external stimuli. This category of neuropsychiatric disturbance includes disinhibition and aggression among other similar problems. These neuropsychiatric disturbances frequently, but not invariably, co-occur with emotional dyscontrol. Although not specific to TBI,[131–133] behavioral dyscontrol is a common, functionally limiting, and treatment-requiring problem among persons with TBI.[47,110] These neuropsychiatric disturbances tend to be more common consequences of moderate or severe TBI rather than mild TBI.[106,134–136]

The DSM-5[59] diagnosis of personality change due to another medical condition applies to these forms of behavioral dyscontrol, with qualifiers for disinhibited type (if the predominant feature is poor impulse control), aggressive type (if the predominant feature is aggressive behavior), or combined type (if more than one of these disturbances predominate the clinical presentation). All of these diagnoses correspond to *DSM-5* and *ICD-9-CM* code 301.1. Posttraumatic aggression may also be assigned *ICD-9-CM* code 301.3, to which the descriptor synonyms *aggressiveness, aggressive reaction, aggressive behavior (finding)*, or *aggressive behavior disorder* apply.

Disinhibition

Disinhibition refers to socially or contextually inappropriate nonaggressive verbal, physical, and sexual acts that reflect a lessening or loss of inhibitions and/or inability to appreciate social or cultural behavioral norms. In the TBI literature, this behavior often is described in association (or synonymously) with impulsivity.[106,134,137–140] However, impulsivity is only one of several characteristics of disinhibition, with others including deficits in patience and frustration tolerance, social cognition, and comportment (ie, the ability to align interpersonal, social, and sexual conduct with social and cultural norms). Although disinhibition and aggression frequently co-occur among persons with TBI,[6,7,118,119] these are distinct categories of behavioral dyscontrol.

Common clinical experience suggests that disinhibition is a relatively frequent problem during the early period following moderate or severe TBI,[10,11] but the prevalence of disinhibition, assessed as such, during this period is not well established. In the late postinjury period, the reported frequencies of disinhibition in clinical samples of persons with moderate to severe TBI range from 12% to 32%.[6,7,87,118,119] The presence and severity of disinhibition is associated with poor long-term outcomes,[6,7] reduced functional independence,[118] and social disability.[141]

The differential diagnosis for disinhibition includes mood disorders (especially bipolar spectrum disorders), psychotic disorders, substance use disorders, personality disorders (especially borderline personality disorder), and other developmental, acquired, and neurodegenerative neurologic conditions. Even when the diagnosis of TBI is unequivocal, these other causes of disinhibited behavior require consideration during the clinical evaluation and in relation to treatment planning.

Among patients with the capacity for reliable self-report, the Barratt Impulsiveness Scale[142] (including a 15-item short form of this measure that assesses nonplanned behavior, motor impulsivity, and attention impulsivity[143]) may provide a framework for characterizing and monitoring disinhibited behavior among persons with TBI.[144] However, this measure is limited as an assessment of disinhibition given its relatively narrow focus on impulsivity, the differential diagnosis for which includes a wide range of neurologic, psychiatric (including personality), and substance use disorders.[143]

Among patients with posttraumatic self-awareness deficits, informant-based assessment will be required to assess disinhibition. The disinhibition subscale of the NPI[68–71] provides a framework for informant-based identification and characterization of this type of behavioral dyscontrol. It includes questions about impulsivity, impatience, social cognitive deficits, and inappropriate interpersonal, social, and sexual behaviors. The NPI-C[71] integrates informant-based and clinician-observed data and is especially useful for the clinical and research evaluation of disinhibition. Once caregivers and other informants are educated about this form of behavioral dyscontrol, the NPI-Q[70] serves usefully as a vehicle for enhancing subsequent clinician-caregiver communications about and monitoring of posttraumatic disinhibition.

The treatment of posttraumatic disinhibition often requires behavioral, environmental, and pharmacologic approaches.[145] Applied behavioral analysis and treatment is a useful element of the treatment plan for disinhibited behaviors.[146–148] This approach entails careful characterization of the disinhibited behaviors, their internal and external (ie, environmental, interpersonal) antecedents, and their consequences (including unintended reinforcers). Social skills training, including individual[149] and group[149–151] interventions, also may be useful. The participation of family members and others with whom individuals with posttraumatic disinhibition interact is an essential component of effective treatment, particularly with regard to ensuring consistency of environmental and behavioral interventions.

The evidence base on which to base pharmacotherapy of posttraumatic disinhibition specifically (ie, separate from posttraumatic aggression) is underdeveloped. However, published treatment approaches used for this purpose in other populations (eg, frontotemporal dementia, neurodevelopmental disorders) may inform selection of treatments for posttraumatic disinhibition. For example, SSRIs decrease behavioral drive and therefore are used to diminish disinhibition in other neurologic conditions, especially frontotemporal dementia.[152–155] When this approach is used to treat posttraumatic disinhibition and associated symptoms of emotional and behavioral dyscontrol, relatively high doses of these medications may be required. Anticonvulsant medications, including valproate, carbamazepine, and lamotrigine,[125,156] are used to reduce disinhibition in a variety of psychiatric and neurologic conditions. Doses used to treat posttraumatic disinhibition are similar to those used in the treatment of secondary mania or posttraumatic epilepsy. There are reports that antiandrogenic agents may reduce sexually impulsive or disinhibited behaviors,[157] although reviews of this approach suggest that it is inconsistently effective and entails complex proxy consent considerations. If all of these approaches fail partially or completely, then adjunctive or primary treatment with atypical antipsychotic agents may be necessary.[158,159]

Agents that augment cerebral catecholaminergic function (ie, stimulants, amantadine) are used to treat posttraumatic cognitive impairments and may concurrently reduce disinhibition.[41,72,138,139] The effectiveness of amantadine for chronic posttraumatic irritability and aggression[47] also offers promise of possible benefits of this agent on posttraumatic disinhibition.

Aggression

In the TBI literature, the term *aggression* has been used to denote many forms of emotional and behavioral dyscontrol, including irritability, anger, agitation, and disinhibition, among others.[24,110,160] For the purposes of this article, the authors limit the referents of aggression to verbal outbursts or physical violence to objects or other people. This form of behavioral dyscontrol places persons with TBI and those around them in harm's way, interferes with rehabilitation, compromises social support networks and is among the most challenging consequences of TBI to manage effectively.[161]

The prototypical form of posttraumatic aggression was described by Yudofsky and Silver[162] (1985) as the "organic aggressive syndrome." This syndrome is characterized by aggression that is reactive (ie, easily provoked), explosive (ie, occurs suddenly and without any apparent buildup), nonreflective (ie, unplanned), noninstrumental (ie, serves no clear long-term aim or objective), periodic (ie, aggressive outbursts occur amid relative calm between episodes), and ego-dystonic. Although useful as a model of posttraumatic aggression, common clinical experience suggests that most presentations of posttraumatic aggression do not conform strictly to this syndrome. The variability in presentations of posttraumatic aggression makes it difficult to establish confidently the causal relationships between TBI and violent acts.

In the service of providing clinicians guidance on these matters, Wortzel and Arciniegas (2013)[160] proposed typologies of posttraumatic aggression modeled on the typologies of violence described by Reid and Thorne (2008).[163] Aggression that is purposeful (ie, reflects intent, premeditation, determination, and/or resolve to act violently) and instrumental (ie, serves as a means to a specific end) falls at the opposite end of the spectrum of posttraumatic aggression from the organic aggression syndrome, which by definition is neither purposeful nor instrumental. Examples of purposeful, instrumental aggression include violence for hire or revenge. This form of aggression is atypical of posttraumatic aggression, posttraumatic only in the sense that it occurs at some point after a (usually remote) TBI, and implausibly framed as a direct consequence of TBI.[160] At midpoints on the dimensions of purposefulness and instrumentality are aggressive behaviors directed at a specific person in response to a perceived (but potentially imagined) threat or that maladaptively serve as a means to a desired end.

Estimates of the frequency of posttraumatic aggression are confounded by variability in the referents of this term, with some studies using other terms as synonyms for aggressive behaviors (ie, *agitation, restlessness, impulsivity, disinhibition, irritability, lability,* or *explosive behaviors*) and others using such terms to denote distinct forms of emotional or behavioral dyscontrol.[160,164] The frequency of aggression (specifically) within the first 6 months following mild TBI has been estimated at 5% to 8% in a sample of military service members, most of who were studied in the first 3 months after injury.[165] In the late period following mild TBI, posttraumatic aggression has been associated with preinjury personality disorders, especially antisocial personality disorder.[166] Importantly, Tateno and colleagues[29] (2003) observed aggression (as assessed by Overt Aggression Scale[131] scores $\geq$3) in 11% of persons without a history of TBI serving as an other injury comparison group in their study of posttraumatic aggression. This observation suggests that interpretation of estimated frequencies of aggression among people with histories of mild TBI require contextualization with trauma experience and other personal variables unrelated to neurotrauma.

Among persons with more severe injuries, early posttraumatic confusional state-related agitation and aggression occurs in 30% to 80%,[16,29,114,167] with as many as 20% demonstrating violent behavior.[114] In the late postinjury period following nonpenetrating severe TBI, rates of aggression range from 15% to 51%.[6,7,29,86,87,118,119] Among studies using the NPI[68] to identify agitation/aggression, the estimated frequency of chronic posttraumatic aggression is approximately 20%.[6,7,29,86,118,119]

Although aggression can be a direct neuropsychiatric consequence of TBI, its development is influenced by preinjury and postinjury comorbidities; these include mood disorders, trauma spectrum disorders, psychotic disorders, personality disorders, substance use disorders, pain, and medications with adverse behavioral effects.[7,23–32,34–36] Depression and anxiety, in particular, are strongly associated with the development of aggression in the late period following TBI[23,24,29] and need to be considered as possible primary diagnoses among people presenting with posttraumatic aggression. When any of these conditions are present in a person with posttraumatic aggression, their treatment may reduce behavioral dyscontrol and obviate treatment targeting posttraumatic aggression specifically.

Among patients with the capacity for accurate self-report, identification of the contexts, frequency, and severity of posttraumatic aggression may be augmented usefully by the administration of the Aggression Questionnaire-12,[168,169] a 12-item self-report measure of physical aggression, verbal aggression, anger, and hostility. The Personality Assessment Inventory,[170] a multidimensional measure, also appears to be useful for the assessment of posttraumatic aggression and co-occurring psychiatric symptoms.[165] Among patients with co-occurring cognitive or self-awareness deficits, the assessment of aggression requires interviewing a knowledgeable informant. When the clinical assessment suggests that symptom-specific assessment will suffice (ie, when concurrent assessment of other neuropsychiatric symptoms is either not necessary or accomplished by coadministration of other scales), the Overt Aggression Scale,[131] Modified Overt Aggression Scale,[171] or the Overt Aggression Scale-Modified for Neurorehabilitation[172] may be used for this purpose. Among these measures, the Modified Overt Aggression Scale is included in the NINDS CDEs for TBI[117] and recommended for these purposes. Alternatively, the NPI[68–71] is useful when multidimensional neuropsychiatric assessment is required and has been used productively to identify the frequency and severity of aggression and co-occurring neuropsychiatric symptoms among persons with TBI.[6,7,47,118,119]

Effective treatment of posttraumatic aggression requires a multimodal, multidisciplinary, collaborative approach and usually involves combined nonpharmacologic and pharmacologic interventions.[110,173] Applied behavioral analysis and behavioral management techniques are useful for the management of aggression among persons with TBI[174] and include replacement strategies and decelerative techniques.[175] Replacement strategies include assertiveness training (intended for patients who become angry when they fail to get their needs met) and differential reinforcement scheduling (to decrease the rate of previolent behaviors). Decelerative techniques include social extinction, contingent observation, self-controlled time-out, overcorrection, and contingent restraint. Wood and Thomas (2013)[173] also suggest that modified forms of cognitive behavioral therapy may be useful for the management of aggression among persons with TBI in a manner analogous to their application for this purpose in other populations.[176–178] Preliminary reports suggest that cognitive behavioral therapy may reduce posttraumatic aggression[169,179,180] and are encouraging of further study of this intervention.

The pharmacotherapy of posttraumatic aggression is conceptually divided into two categories: interventions for acute aggression and treatments for chronic aggression. Antipsychotics and benzodiazepines are the most commonly used medications in the treatment of acute aggressive, agitated, and self-injurious behaviors among persons with TBI.[181–183] However, their use among persons with TBI may reduce the rate of recovery and produce adverse cognitive and motor effects during the early postinjury period.[36,184] Accordingly, the use of these agents needs to be weighed against the risks of harm to self and others as well as the risk of reinjury or medical complications associated with uncontrolled aggression. If antipsychotics are used to treat acute aggression, then atypical (ie, second-generation) antipsychotics, such as quetiapine, olanzapine, or aripiprazole, are preferred in light of their relatively favorable adverse cognitive and motor side-effect profiles. When these agents are used, low and frequent dosing with rapid dose titration to effectiveness and/or sedation is the recommended approach. If an atypical antipsychotic is not effective, then low-dose haloperidol prescribed according to a similar dose-escalation protocol is a reasonable alternative treatment of acute aggression.[185] When this medication is used, monitoring for treatment-related akathisia and extrapyramidal side effects and distinguishing these from treatment-refractory agitation and aggression is essential in order to avoid initiating a cycle of continued dose escalation and behavioral deterioration. If benzodiazepines must be used adjunctively to reduce acute aggression, using serum metabolized agents with short- or moderate-duration half-lives and no active metabolites (eg, lorazepam, oxazepam) is suggested.

When acute aggression abates, doses of antipsychotics (and, if used, benzodiazepines) are decreased gradually and, whenever possible, discontinued. Chronic treatment with antipsychotics is usually reserved for patients with persistent psychotic symptoms or chronic aggression refractory to treatment with other medications. Chronic treatment with benzodiazepines should be avoided.

Chronic aggression often requires long-term symptom-targeted pharmacotherapy. Treatment must be coupled with realistic treatment goals; in many cases, it may not be possible to eliminate posttraumatic aggression, and a more appropriate (and achievable) goal is reducing the frequency and severity of aggressive behaviors. The Neurobehavioral Guidelines Working Group[37] concluded that the evidence is sufficient to support the use of serotonin reuptake inhibitors, tricyclic antidepressants, buspirone, methylphenidate, valproate, lithium, or the beta-adrenergic receptor antagonists propranolol or pindolol for the treatment of chronic posttraumatic aggression. Among these medications, the best evidence was for the beta-adrenergic receptor antagonists; in clinical practice, however, these agents are generally reserved for use among patients who fail to respond to other medications.

Among individuals with relatively preserved dorsal and lateral prefrontal areas capable of effecting top-down modulation of behavior, augmenting the function of these brain areas (and the behavior-regulating circuits to which they contribute) with amantadine, methylphenidate, dextroamphetamine, and bromocriptine may reduce agitated, aggressive, and/or self-injurious behaviors. When behavioral dyscontrol is thought to reflect diminished top-down regulation of ventral brain structures driving aggressive behavior, using medications that reduce limbic catecholaminergic function (ie, atypical antipsychotics or beta-adrenergic receptor antagonists) or that attenuate activity in those structures (ie, SSRIs, atypical antipsychotics, anticonvulsants, or un-competitive N-methyl-D-aspartate receptor antagonists such as amantadine) may be useful. In clinical practice, SSRIs are a first-line intervention for chronic posttraumatic aggression. Recent evidence suggests that amantadine may also be a useful first-line treatment of this problem.[47] If SSRIs or amantadine are ineffective, the next step in treatment is an anticonvulsant, usually valproate or carbamazepine. Adjunctive treatment with lithium, buspirone, and beta-adrenergic receptor antagonists may be used if SSRIs and anticonvulsants are ineffective or only partially effective. If posttraumatic aggression proves refractory to other interventions, then chronic treatment with atypical antipsychotics may be required and useful.[126,186,187]

SUMMARY

Emotional and behavioral dyscontrol are relatively common and disabling consequences of TBI. Managing these problems effectively requires clinicians to understand their phenomenology and epidemiology. Their assessment is facilitated by the use of valid and reliable symptom-specific and multidimensional neuropsychiatric metrics. Emotional and behavioral dyscontrol frequently co-occur with other posttraumatic neuropsychiatric disturbances, the treatment of which may concurrently reduce the frequency and severity of dyscontrol symptoms. However, when emotional and/or behavioral dyscontrol require symptom-specific treatments, a combination of non-pharmacologic (ie, psychological, behavioral, environmental) and pharmacologic approaches is usually required. When properly administered, these interventions may provide persons with TBI and their families with substantial relief from posttraumatic emotional and behavioral dyscontrol.

REFERENCES

1. Arciniegas DB, Zasler ND, Vanderploeg RD, et al. Management of adults with traumatic brain injury. Washington, DC: American Psychiatric Publishing, Inc; 2013.

2. Silver JM, McAllister TW, Yudofsky SC. Textbook of traumatic brain injury. 2nd edition. Arlington (VA): American Psychiatric Pub; 2011.
3. Levin HS. Neurobehavioral outcome of closed head injury: implications for clinical trials. J Neurotrauma 1995;12(4):601–10.
4. Rapoport M, McCauley S, Levin H, et al. The role of injury severity in neurobehavioral outcome 3 months after traumatic brain injury. Neuropsychiatry Neuropsychol Behav Neurol 2002;15(2):123–32.
5. Hart T, Whyte J, Polansky M, et al. Concordance of patient and family report of neurobehavioral symptoms at 1 year after traumatic brain injury. Arch Phys Med Rehabil 2003;84(2):204–13.
6. Ciurli P, Formisano R, Bivona U, et al. Neuropsychiatric disorders in persons with severe traumatic brain injury: prevalence, phenomenology, and relationship with demographic, clinical, and functional features. J Head Trauma Rehabil 2011; 26(2):116–26.
7. Castano Monsalve B, Bernabeu Guitart M, Lopez R, et al. Psychopathological evaluation of traumatic brain injury patients with the Neuropsychiatric Inventory. Rev Psiquiatr Salud Ment 2012;5(3):160–6.
8. Guilmette TJ, Paglia MF. The public's misconception about traumatic brain injury: a follow up survey. Arch Clin Neuropsychol 2004;19(2):183–9.
9. Swift TL, Wilson SL. Misconceptions about brain injury among the general public and non-expert health professionals: an exploratory study. Brain Inj 2001;15(2): 149–65.
10. Arciniegas DB. Addressing neuropsychiatric disturbances during rehabilitation after traumatic brain injury: current and future methods. Dialogues Clin Neurosci 2011;13(3):325–45.
11. Arciniegas DB, McAllister TW. Neurobehavioral management of traumatic brain injury in the critical care setting. Crit Care Clin 2008;24(4):737–65, viii.
12. Povlishock JT, Katz DI. Update of neuropathology and neurological recovery after traumatic brain injury. J Head Trauma Rehabil 2005;20(1):76–94.
13. Wallesch CW, Curio N, Kutz S, et al. Outcome after mild-to-moderate blunt head injury: effects of focal lesions and diffuse axonal injury. Brain Inj 2001;15(5): 401–12.
14. Wallesch CW, Curio N, Galazky I, et al. The neuropsychology of blunt head injury in the early postacute stage: effects of focal lesions and diffuse axonal injury. J Neurotrauma 2001;18(1):11–20.
15. Nakase-Thompson R, Sherer M, Yablon SA, et al. Acute confusion following traumatic brain injury. Brain Inj 2004;18(2):131–42.
16. Sherer M, Nakase-Thompson R, Yablon SA, et al. Multidimensional assessment of acute confusion after traumatic brain injury. Arch Phys Med Rehabil 2005; 86(5):896–904.
17. Dikmen SS, Machamer JE, Powell JM, et al. Outcome 3 to 5 years after moderate to severe traumatic brain injury. Arch Phys Med Rehabil 2003;84(10): 1449–57.
18. Draper K, Ponsford J, Schonberger M. Psychosocial and emotional outcomes 10 years following traumatic brain injury. J Head Trauma Rehabil 2007;22(5): 278–87.
19. van der Naalt J, van Zomeren AH, Sluiter WJ, et al. Acute behavioural disturbances related to imaging studies and outcome in mild-to-moderate head injury. Brain Inj 2000;14(9):781–8.
20. American Psychiatric Association DSM-5 Task Force. Major or mild neurocognitive disorder due to traumatic brain injury. In: American Psychiatric Association

DSM-5 Task Force, editor. Diagnostic and statistical manual of mental disorders: DSM-5. Washington, DC: American Psychiatric Association; 2013. p. 624–7.
21. Vos PE, Alekseenko Y, Battistin L, et al. Mild traumatic brain injury. Eur J Neurol 2012;19(2):191–8.
22. Carroll LJ, Cassidy JD, Peloso PM, et al. Prognosis for mild traumatic brain injury: results of the WHO Collaborating Centre Task Force on Mild Traumatic Brain Injury. J Rehabil Med 2004;(Suppl 43):84–105.
23. Jorge RE, Robinson RG, Moser D, et al. Major depression following traumatic brain injury. Arch Gen Psychiatry 2004;61(1):42–50.
24. Baguley IJ, Cooper J, Felmingham K. Aggressive behavior following traumatic brain injury: how common is common? J Head Trauma Rehabil 2006;21(1): 45–56.
25. Fann JR, Uomoto JM, Katon WJ. Sertraline in the treatment of major depression following mild traumatic brain injury. J Neuropsychiatry Clin Neurosci 2000; 12(2):226–32.
26. Linn RT, Allen K, Willer BS. Affective symptoms in the chronic stage of traumatic brain injury: a study of married couples. Brain Inj 1994;8(2):135–47.
27. Rao V, Rosenberg P, Bertrand M, et al. Aggression after traumatic brain injury: prevalence and correlates. J Neuropsychiatry Clin Neurosci 2009;21(4): 420–9.
28. Seel RT, Macciocchi S, Kreutzer JS. Clinical considerations for the diagnosis of major depression after moderate to severe TBI. J Head Trauma Rehabil 2010; 25(2):99–112.
29. Tateno A, Jorge RE, Robinson RG. Clinical correlates of aggressive behavior after traumatic brain injury. J Neuropsychiatry Clin Neurosci 2003;15(2):155–60.
30. Johansson SH, Jamora CW, Ruff RM, et al. A biopsychosocial perspective of aggression in the context of traumatic brain injury. Brain Inj 2008;22(13–14): 999–1006.
31. Halbauer JD, Ashford JW, Zeitzer JM, et al. Neuropsychiatric diagnosis and management of chronic sequelae of war-related mild to moderate traumatic brain injury. J Rehabil Res Dev 2009;46(6):757–96.
32. Maguen S, Lau KM, Madden E, et al. Relationship of screen-based symptoms for mild traumatic brain injury and mental health problems in Iraq and Afghanistan veterans: distinct or overlapping symptoms? J Rehabil Res Dev 2012;49(7):1115–26.
33. Silver JM, McAllister TW, Arciniegas DB. Depression and cognitive complaints following mild traumatic brain injury. Am J Psychiatry 2009;166(6):653–61.
34. Weyer Jamora C, Schroeder SC, Ruff RM. Pain and mild traumatic brain injury: the implications of pain severity on emotional and cognitive functioning. Brain Inj 2013;27(10):1134–40.
35. Flanagan SR, Elovic EP, Sandel E. Managing agitation associated with traumatic brain injury: behavioral versus pharmacologic interventions? PM R 2009;1(1): 76–80.
36. Mysiw WJ, Bogner JA, Corrigan JD, et al. The impact of acute care medications on rehabilitation outcome after traumatic brain injury. Brain Inj 2006;20(9): 905–11.
37. Warden DL, Gordon B, McAllister TW, et al. Guidelines for the pharmacologic treatment of neurobehavioral sequelae of traumatic brain injury. J Neurotrauma 2006;23(10):1468–501.
38. Arciniegas DB, Silver JM. Pharmacotherapy of posttraumatic cognitive impairments. Behav Neurol 2006;17(1):25–42.

39. Chew E, Zafonte RD. Pharmacological management of neurobehavioral disorders following traumatic brain injury–a state-of-the-art review. J Rehabil Res Dev 2009;46(6):851–79.
40. Wheaton P, Mathias JL, Vink R. Impact of early pharmacological treatment on cognitive and behavioral outcome after traumatic brain injury in adults: a meta-analysis. J Clin Psychopharmacol 2009;29(5):468–77.
41. Wheaton P, Mathias JL, Vink R. Impact of pharmacological treatments on cognitive and behavioral outcome in the postacute stages of adult traumatic brain injury: a meta-analysis. J Clin Psychopharmacol 2011;31(6):745–57.
42. Cicerone KD, Dahlberg C, Kalmar K, et al. Evidence-based cognitive rehabilitation: recommendations for clinical practice. Arch Phys Med Rehabil 2000; 81(12):1596–615.
43. Cicerone KD, Dahlberg C, Malec JF, et al. Evidence-based cognitive rehabilitation: updated review of the literature from 1998 through 2002. Arch Phys Med Rehabil 2005;86(8):1681–92.
44. Cicerone KD, Langenbahn DM, Braden C, et al. Evidence-based cognitive rehabilitation: updated review of the literature from 2003 through 2008. Arch Phys Med Rehabil 2011;92(4):519–30.
45. Cappa SF, Benke T, Clarke S, et al. EFNS guidelines on cognitive rehabilitation: report of an EFNS task force. Eur J Neurol 2005;12(9):665–80.
46. Cappa SF, Benke T, Clarke S, et al. EFNS guidelines on cognitive rehabilitation: report of an EFNS task force. Eur J Neurol 2003;10(1):11–23.
47. Hammond FM, Bickett AK, Norton JH, et al. Effectiveness of amantadine hydrochloride in the reduction of chronic traumatic brain injury irritability and aggression. J Head Trauma Rehabil 2013. [Epub ahead of print].
48. Arciniegas DB, Topkoff J. The neuropsychiatry of pathologic affect: an approach to evaluation and treatment. Semin Clin Neuropsychiatry 2000;5(4):290–306.
49. Wortzel HS, Oster TJ, Anderson CA, et al. Pathological laughing and crying: epidemiology, pathophysiology and treatment. CNS Drugs 2008;22(7):531–45.
50. Arciniegas DB, Topkoff J, Silver JM. Neuropsychiatric aspects of traumatic brain injury. Curr Treat Options Neurol 2000;2(2):169–86.
51. Tateno A, Jorge RE, Robinson RG. Pathological laughing and crying following traumatic brain injury. J Neuropsychiatry Clin Neurosci 2004;16(4):426–34.
52. Chahine LM, Chemali Z. Du rire aux larmes: pathological laughing and crying in patients with traumatic brain injury and treatment with lamotrigine. Epilepsy Behav 2006;8(3):610–5.
53. Cummings JL, Arciniegas DB, Brooks BR, et al. Defining and diagnosing involuntary emotional expression disorder. CNS Spectr 2006;11(6):1–7.
54. McGrath J. A study of emotionalism in patients undergoing rehabilitation following severe acquired brain injury. Behav Neurol 2000;12(4):201–7.
55. Muller U, Murai T, Bauer-Wittmund T, et al. Paroxetine versus citalopram treatment of pathological crying after brain injury. Brain Inj 1999;13(10):805–11.
56. Sloan RL, Brown KW, Pentland B. Fluoxetine as a treatment for emotional lability after brain injury. Brain Inj 1992;6(4):315–9.
57. Zeilig G, Drubach DA, Katz-Zeilig M, et al. Pathological laughter and crying in patients with closed traumatic brain injury. Brain Inj 1996;10(8):591–7.
58. Tate RL. Executive dysfunction and characterological changes after traumatic brain injury: two sides of the same coin? Cortex 1999;35(1):39–55.
59. American Psychiatric Association DSM-5 Task Force. Diagnostic and statistical manual of mental disorders: DSM-5. 5th edition. Washington, DC: American Psychiatric Association; 2013.

60. National Center for Health Statistics. International classification of diseases. 9th edition. Atlanta (GA): Centers for Disease Control and Prevention; 2009. Clinical Modification.
61. Wilson SA. Some problems in neurology: no. II - pathological laughing and crying. J Neurol Psychopathol 1924;4(16):299–333.
62. Olney NT, Goodkind MS, Lomen-Hoerth C, et al. Behaviour, physiology and experience of pathological laughing and crying in amyotrophic lateral sclerosis. Brain 2011;134(Pt 12):3458–69.
63. Lauterbach EC, Cummings JL, Kuppuswamy PS. Toward a more precise, clinically–informed pathophysiology of pathological laughing and crying. Neurosci Biobehav Rev 2013;37(8):1893–916.
64. Rabins PV, Arciniegas DB. Pathophysiology of involuntary emotional expression disorder. CNS Spectr 2007;12(4 Suppl 5):17–22.
65. Robinson RG, Parikh RM, Lipsey JR, et al. Pathological laughing and crying following stroke: validation of a measurement scale and a double-blind treatment study. Am J Psychiatry 1993;150(2):286–93.
66. Green RL, McAllister TW, Bernat JL. A study of crying in medically and surgically hospitalized patients. Am J Psychiatry 1987;144(4):442–7.
67. Moore SR, Gresham LS, Bromberg MB, et al. A self report measure of affective lability. J Neurol Neurosurg Psychiatr 1997;63(1):89–93.
68. Cummings JL, Mega M, Gray K, et al. The Neuropsychiatric Inventory: comprehensive assessment of psychopathology in dementia. Neurology 1994;44(12):2308–14.
69. Wood S, Cummings JL, Hsu MA, et al. The use of the neuropsychiatric inventory in nursing home residents. Characterization and measurement. Am J Geriatr Psychiatry 2000;8(1):75–83.
70. Kaufer DI, Cummings JL, Ketchel P, et al. Validation of the NPI-Q, a brief clinical form of the Neuropsychiatric Inventory. J Neuropsychiatry Clin Neurosci 2000; 12(2):233–9.
71. de Medeiros K, Robert P, Gauthier S, et al. The Neuropsychiatric Inventory-Clinician rating scale (NPI-C): reliability and validity of a revised assessment of neuropsychiatric symptoms in dementia. Int Psychogeriatr 2010;22(6):984–94.
72. Evans RW, Gualtieri CT, Patterson D. Treatment of chronic closed head injury with psychostimulant drugs: a controlled case study and an appropriate evaluation procedure. J Nerv Ment Dis 1987;175(2):106–10.
73. Udaka F, Yamao S, Nagata H, et al. Pathologic laughing and crying treated with levodopa. Arch Neurol 1984;41(10):1095–6.
74. Lewin J, Sumners D. Successful treatment of episodic dyscontrol with carbamazepine. Br J Psychiatry 1992;161:261–2.
75. Poeck K. Pathophysiology of emotional disorders associated with brain damage. Handbook of Clinical Neurology 1969;3:343–67.
76. Siever LJ, Davis KL. A psychobiological perspective on the personality disorders. Am J Psychiatry 1991;148(12):1647–58.
77. Henry C, Van den Bulke D, Bellivier F, et al. Affective lability and affect intensity as core dimensions of bipolar disorders during euthymic period. Psychiatry Res 2008;159(1–2):1–6.
78. Beresford TP, Arciniegas D, Clapp L, et al. Reduction of affective lability and alcohol use following traumatic brain injury: a clinical pilot study of anticonvulsant medications. Brain Inj 2005;19(4):309–13.
79. Woyshville MJ, Lackamp JM, Eisengart JA, et al. On the meaning and measurement of affective instability: clues from chaos theory. Biol Psychiatry 1999;45(3): 261–9.

80. Villemure R, Nolin P, Le Sage N. Self-reported symptoms during post-mild traumatic brain injury in acute phase: influence of interviewing method. Brain Inj 2011;25(1):53–64.
81. King NS, Crawford S, Wenden FJ, et al. The Rivermead Post Concussion Symptoms Questionnaire: a measure of symptoms commonly experienced after head injury and its reliability. J Neurol 1995;242(9):587–92.
82. Cicerone K, Kalmar K. Persistent postconcussion syndrome: the structure of subjective complaints after mild traumatic brain injury. J Head Trauma Rehabil 1995;10:1–17.
83. Meterko M, Baker E, Stolzmann KL, et al. Psychometric assessment of the Neurobehavioral Symptom Inventory-22: the structure of persistent postconcussive symptoms following deployment-related mild traumatic brain injury among veterans. J Head Trauma Rehabil 2012;27(1):55–62.
84. Kreutzer JS, Marwitz JH, Seel R, et al. Validation of a neurobehavioral functioning inventory for adults with traumatic brain injury. Arch Phys Med Rehabil 1996;77(2):116–24.
85. McKinlay WW, Brooks DN, Bond MR, et al. The short-term outcome of severe blunt head injury as reported by relatives of the injured persons. J Neurol Neurosurg Psychiatr 1981;44(6):527–33.
86. Pelegrin-Valero CA, Gomez-Hernandez R, Munoz-Cespedes JM, et al. Nosologic aspects of personality change due to head trauma. Rev Neurol 2001;32(7):681–7.
87. Deb S, Lyons I, Koutzoukis C. Neurobehavioural symptoms one year after a head injury. Br J Psychiatry 1999;174:360–5.
88. Harvey PD, Greenberg BR, Serper MR. The affective lability scales: development, reliability, and validity. J Clin Psychol 1989;45(5):786–93.
89. Solhan MB, Trull TJ, Jahng S, et al. Clinical assessment of affective instability: comparing EMA indices, questionnaire reports, and retrospective recall. Psychol Assess 2009;21(3):425–36.
90. Mackinnon DF, Pies R. Affective instability as rapid cycling: theoretical and clinical implications for borderline personality and bipolar spectrum disorders. Bipolar Disord 2006;8(1):1–14.
91. Parmentier C, Etain B, Yon L, et al. Clinical and dimensional characteristics of euthymic bipolar patients with or without suicidal behavior. Eur Psychiatry 2012;27(8):570–6.
92. Henry C, Mitropoulou V, New AS, et al. Affective instability and impulsivity in borderline personality and bipolar II disorders: similarities and differences. J Psychiatr Res 2001;35(6):307–12.
93. Reich DB, Zanarini MC, Bieri KA. A preliminary study of lamotrigine in the treatment of affective instability in borderline personality disorder. Int Clin Psychopharmacol 2009;24(5):270–5.
94. Koenigsberg HW, Harvey PD, Mitropoulou V, et al. Characterizing affective instability in borderline personality disorder. Am J Psychiatry 2002;159(5):784–8.
95. Look AE, Flory JD, Harvey PD, et al. Psychometric properties of a short form of the Affective Lability Scale (ALS-18). Pers Individ Dif 2010;49(3):187–91.
96. Block SH. Psychotherapy of the individual with brain injury. Brain Inj 1987;1(2):203–6.
97. Wilson BA. Neuropsychological rehabilitation. Annu Rev Clin Psychol 2008;4:141–62.
98. Leon Carrion J, Machuca Murga F, Murga Sierra M, et al. Outcome after an intensive, holistic and multidisciplinary rehabilitation program after traumatic brain injury. Medico legal values. Rev Neurol 2001;33(4):377–83.

99. Cicerone KD, Mott T, Azulay J, et al. A randomized controlled trial of holistic neuropsychologic rehabilitation after traumatic brain injury. Arch Phys Med Rehabil 2008;89(12):2239–49.
100. Caracuel A, Cuberos-Urbano G, Santiago-Ramajo S, et al. Effectiveness of holistic neuropsychological rehabilitation for Spanish population with acquired brain injury measured using Rasch analysis. NeuroRehabilitation 2012;30(1): 43–53.
101. Cattelani R, Zettin M, Zoccolotti P. Rehabilitation treatments for adults with behavioral and psychosocial disorders following acquired brain injury: a systematic review. Neuropsychol Rev 2010;20(1):52–85.
102. Scherer KR, Wranik T, Sangsue J, et al. Emotions in everyday life: probability and occurrence, risk factors, appraisal, and reaction patterns. Soc Sci Inf 2004;43(4): 499–570.
103. Yang CC, Huang SJ, Lin WC, et al. Divergent manifestations of irritability in patients with mild and moderate-to-severe traumatic brain injury: perspectives of awareness and neurocognitive correlates. Brain Inj 2013;27(9):1008–15.
104. Ettenhofer ML, Abeles N. The significance of mild traumatic brain injury to cognition and self-reported symptoms in long-term recovery from injury. J Clin Exp Neuropsychol 2009;31(3):363–72.
105. Ettenhofer ML, Barry DM. A comparison of long-term postconcussive symptoms between university students with and without a history of mild traumatic brain injury or orthopedic injury. J Int Neuropsychol Soc 2012;18(3):451–60.
106. Bohnen N, Twijnstra A, Jolles J. Post-traumatic and emotional symptoms in different subgroups of patients with mild head injury. Brain Inj 1992;6(6): 481–7.
107. Dikmen S, McLean A, Temkin N. Neuropsychological and psychosocial consequences of minor head injury. J Neurol Neurosurg Psychiatr 1986;49(11): 1227–32.
108. van der Naalt J, van Zomeren AH, Sluiter WJ, et al. One year outcome in mild to moderate head injury: the predictive value of acute injury characteristics related to complaints and return to work. J Neurol Neurosurg Psychiatr 1999;66(2): 207–13.
109. Kim SH, Manes F, Kosier T, et al. Irritability following traumatic brain injury. J Nerv Ment Dis 1999;187(6):327–35.
110. Alderman N. Contemporary approaches to the management of irritability and aggression following traumatic brain injury. Neuropsychol Rehabil 2003;13(1–2): 211–40.
111. Eames PG. Distinguishing the neuropsychiatric, psychiatric, and psychological consequences of acquired brain injury. In: Wood RL, McMillan T, editors. Neurobehavioral disability and social handicap following traumatic brain injury. Hove (United Kingdom): Psychology Press; 2001. p. 29–46.
112. Iverson GL, McCracken LM. 'Postconcussive' symptoms in persons with chronic pain. Brain Inj 1997;11(11):783–90.
113. Yang CC, Hua MS, Lin WC, et al. Irritability following traumatic brain injury: divergent manifestations of annoyance and verbal aggression. Brain Inj 2012;26(10): 1185–91.
114. Brooks DN, McKinlay WW, Symington C, et al. The effects of severe head injury upon patient and relative within seven years of injury. J Head Trauma Rehabil 1987;2:1–13.
115. Craig KJ, Hietanen H, Markova IS, et al. The Irritability Questionnaire: a new scale for the measurement of irritability. Psychiatry Res 2008;159(3):367–75.

116. Yang CC, Huang SJ, Lin WC, et al. Evaluating irritability in patients with traumatic brain injury: development of the National Taiwan University Irritability Scale. Brain Impair 2011;12:200–9.
117. National Institute of Neurologic Disorders and Stroke Common Data Elements Team. Traumatic brain injury common data elements, version 2.01. 2013. Available at: http://www.commondataelements.ninds.nih.gov/tbi.aspx#tab=Data_Standards. Accessed June 27, 2013.
118. Cantagallo A, DiMarco F. Prevalence of neuropsychiatric disorders in traumatic brain injury patients. Eur Med 2002;38(4):167–78.
119. Kilmer RP, Demakis GJ, Hammond FM, et al. Use of the Neuropsychiatric Inventory in traumatic brain injury: a pilot investigation. Rehabil Psychol 2006;51(3):232–8.
120. Rees RJ, Bellon ML. Post concussion syndrome ebb and flow: longitudinal effects and management. NeuroRehabilitation 2007;22(3):229–42.
121. Hart T, Vaccaro MJ, Hays C, et al. Anger self-management training for people with traumatic brain injury: a preliminary investigation. J Head Trauma Rehabil 2012;27(2):113–22.
122. Walker AJ, Nott MT, Doyle M, et al. Effectiveness of a group anger management programme after severe traumatic brain injury. Brain Inj 2010;24(3):517–24.
123. Kant R, Smith-Seemiller L, Zeiler D. Treatment of aggression and irritability after head injury. Brain Inj 1998;12(8):661–6.
124. Wroblewski BA, Joseph AB, Kupfer J, et al. Effectiveness of valproic acid on destructive and aggressive behaviours in patients with acquired brain injury. Brain Inj 1997;11(1):37–47.
125. Azouvi P, Jokic C, Attal N, et al. Carbamazepine in agitation and aggressive behaviour following severe closed-head injury: results of an open trial. Brain Inj 1999;13(10):797–804.
126. Kim E, Bijlani M. A pilot study of quetiapine treatment of aggression due to traumatic brain injury. J Neuropsychiatry Clin Neurosci 2006;18(4):547–9.
127. Umene-Nakano W, Yoshimura R, Okamoto T, et al. Aripiprazole improves various cognitive and behavioral impairments after traumatic brain injury: a case report. Gen Hosp Psychiatry 2013;35(1):103.e7–9.
128. Gualtieri CT. Buspirone: neuropsychiatric effects. J Head Trauma Rehabil 1991;6:90–2.
129. Elliott FA. Propranolol for the control of belligerent behavior following acute brain damage. Ann Neurol 1977;1(5):489–91.
130. Chapman EH, Weintraub RJ, Milburn MA, et al. Homeopathic treatment of mild traumatic brain injury: a randomized, double-blind, placebo-controlled clinical trial. J Head Trauma Rehabil 1999;14(6):521–42.
131. Yudofsky SC, Silver JM, Jackson W, et al. The Overt Aggression Scale for the objective rating of verbal and physical aggression. Am J Psychiatry 1986;143(1):35–9.
132. Fava M. Psychopharmacologic treatment of pathologic aggression. Psychiatr Clin North Am 1997;20(2):427–51.
133. Arciniegas DB, Anderson CA, Filley CM. Behavioral neurology & neuropsychiatry. Cambridge (United Kingdom): Cambridge University Press; 2013.
134. Levin HS, Grossman RG. Behavioral sequelae of closed head injury. A quantitative study. Arch Neurol 1978;35(11):720–7.
135. Max JE, Castillo CS, Bokura H, et al. Oppositional defiant disorder symptomatology after traumatic brain injury: a prospective study. J Nerv Ment Dis 1998;186(6):325–32.

136. Kolitz BP, Vanderploeg RD, Curtiss G. Development of the Key Behaviors Change Inventory: a traumatic brain injury behavioral outcome assessment instrument. Arch Phys Med Rehabil 2003;84(2):277–84.

137. Thomsen IV. Late outcome of very severe blunt head trauma: a 10–15 year second follow-up. J Neurol Neurosurg Psychiatr 1984;47(3):260–8.

138. Kraus MF, Maki PM. Effect of amantadine hydrochloride on symptoms of frontal lobe dysfunction in brain injury: case studies and review. J Neuropsychiatry Clin Neurosci 1997;9(2):222–30.

139. Kraus MF, Maki P. The combined use of amantadine and l-dopa/carbidopa in the treatment of chronic brain injury. Brain Inj 1997;11(6):455–60.

140. McAllister TW. Neuropsychiatric sequelae of head injuries. Psychiatr Clin North Am 1992;15(2):395–413.

141. Dahlberg C, Hawley L, Morey C, et al. Social communication skills in persons with post-acute traumatic brain injury: three perspectives. Brain Inj 2006; 20(4):425–35.

142. Barratt ES. Anxiety and impulsiveness related to psychomotor efficiency. Percept Mot Skills 1959;9:191–8.

143. Spinella M. Normative data and a short form of the Barratt Impulsiveness Scale. Int J Neurosci 2007;117(3):359–68.

144. Votruba KL, Rapport LJ, Vangel SJ Jr, et al. Impulsivity and traumatic brain injury: the relations among behavioral observation, performance measures, and rating scales. J Head Trauma Rehabil 2008;23(2):65–73.

145. Kim E. Agitation, aggression, and disinhibition syndromes after traumatic brain injury. NeuroRehabilitation 2002;17(4):297–310.

146. Karol RL. Principles of applied behavioral analysis and treatment. In: Zasler ND, Katz DI, Zafonte RD, editors. Brain injury medicine: principles and practice. 2nd edition. New York: Demos Medical Publishing; 2013. p. 1053–66.

147. Flashman LA, McAllister TW. Environmental and behavioral interventions. In: Arciniegas DB, Anderson CA, Filley CM, editors. Behavioral neurology & neuropsychiatry. Cambridge (United Kingdom): Cambridge University Press; 2013. p. 604–26.

148. Yody BB, Schaub C, Conway J, et al. Applied behavior management and acquired brain injury: approaches and assessment. J Head Trauma Rehabil 2000;15(4):1041–60.

149. McDonald S, Tate R, Togher L, et al. Social skills treatment for people with severe, chronic acquired brain injuries: a multicenter trial. Arch Phys Med Rehabil 2008;89(9):1648–59.

150. Dahlberg CA, Cusick CP, Hawley LA, et al. Treatment efficacy of social communication skills training after traumatic brain injury: a randomized treatment and deferred treatment controlled trial. Arch Phys Med Rehabil 2007;88(12): 1561–73.

151. Braden C, Hawley L, Newman J, et al. Social communication skills group treatment: a feasibility study for persons with traumatic brain injury and comorbid conditions. Brain Inj 2010;24(11):1298–310.

152. Chow TW. Treatment approaches to symptoms associated with frontotemporal degeneration. Curr Psychiatry Rep 2005;7(5):376–80.

153. Mendez MF. Frontotemporal dementia: therapeutic interventions. Front Neurol Neurosci 2009;24:168–78.

154. Swartz JR, Miller BL, Lesser IM, et al. Frontotemporal dementia: treatment response to serotonin selective reuptake inhibitors. J Clin Psychiatry 1997; 58(5):212–6.

155. Herrmann N, Black SE, Chow T, et al. Serotonergic function and treatment of behavioral and psychological symptoms of frontotemporal dementia. Am J Geriatr Psychiatry 2012;20(9):789–97.

156. Ripoll LH. Clinical psychopharmacology of borderline personality disorder: an update on the available evidence in light of the Diagnostic and Statistical Manual of Mental Disorders - 5. Curr Opin Psychiatry 2012;25(1):52–8.

157. Guay DR. Drug treatment of paraphilic and nonparaphilic sexual disorders. Clin Ther 2009;31(1):1–31.

158. Elovic EP, Jasey NN Jr, Eisenberg ME. The use of atypical antipsychotics after traumatic brain injury. J Head Trauma Rehabil 2008;23(2):132–5.

159. Sink KM, Holden KF, Yaffe K. Pharmacological treatment of neuropsychiatric symptoms of dementia: a review of the evidence. JAMA 2005;293(5):596–608.

160. Wortzel HS, Arciniegas DB. A forensic neuropsychiatric approach to traumatic brain injury, aggression, and suicide. J Am Acad Psychiatry Law 2013;41(2):274–86.

161. Hall KM, Karzmark P, Stevens M, et al. Family stressors in traumatic brain injury: a two-year follow-up. Arch Phys Med Rehabil 1994;75(8):876–84.

162. Yudofsky SC, Silver JM. Psychiatric aspects of brain injury: trauma, stroke, and tumor. In: Hales RE, Frances AJ, editors. American Psychiatric Association Annual Review, vol. 4. Washington, DC: American Psychiatric Press; 1985. p. 142–58.

163. Reid WH, Thorne SA. Personality disorders. In: Simon RI, Tardiff K, editors. Textbook of violence assessment and management. Arlington (VA): American Psychiatric Publishing, Inc; 2008. p. 161–84.

164. Kim E, Lauterbach EC, Reeve A, et al. Neuropsychiatric complications of traumatic brain injury: a critical review of the literature (a report by the ANPA Committee on Research). J Neuropsychiatry Clin Neurosci 2007;19(2):106–27.

165. Lange RT, Brickell TA, French LM, et al. Neuropsychological outcome from uncomplicated mild, complicated mild, and moderate traumatic brain injury in US military personnel. Arch Clin Neuropsychol 2012;27(5):480–94.

166. Ferguson SD, Coccaro EF. History of mild to moderate traumatic brain injury and aggression in physically healthy participants with and without personality disorder. J Personal Disord 2009;23(3):230–9.

167. Eames PE, Wood RL. Episodic disorders of behaviour and affect after acquired brain injury. Neuropsychol Rehabil 2003;13(1–2):241–58.

168. Bryant FB, Smith BD. Refining the architecture of aggression: a measurement model for the Buss-Perry Aggression Questionnaire. J Res Pers 2001;35(2):138–67.

169. Aboulafia-Brakha T, Greber Buschbeck C, Rochat L, et al. Feasibility and initial efficacy of a cognitive-behavioural group programme for managing anger and aggressiveness after traumatic brain injury. Neuropsychol Rehabil 2013;23(2):216–33.

170. Morey LC. Personality assessment inventory: professional manual. Odessa (FL): Psychological Assessment Resources; 1991.

171. Sorgi P, Ratey J, Knoedler DW, et al. Rating aggression in the clinical setting. A retrospective adaptation of the Overt Aggression Scale: preliminary results. J Neuropsychiatry Clin Neurosci 1991;3(2):S52–6.

172. Alderman N, Knight C, Morgan C. Use of a modified version of the Overt Aggression Scale in the measurement and assessment of aggressive behaviours following brain injury. Brain Inj 1997;11(7):503–23.

173. Wood RL, Thomas RH. Impulsive and episodic disorders of aggressive behaviour following traumatic brain injury. Brain Inj 2013;27(3):253–61.

174. Wood RL, Alderman N. Applications of operant learning theory to the management of challenging behavior after traumatic brain injury. J Head Trauma Rehabil 2011;26(3):202–11.
175. Corrigan JD, Bogner J, Lamb-Hart G, et al. Increasing substance abuse treatment compliance for persons with traumatic brain injury. Psychol Addict Behav 2005;19(2):131–9.
176. Willner P, Rose J, Jahoda A, et al. Group-based cognitive-behavioural anger management for people with mild to moderate intellectual disabilities: cluster randomised controlled trial. Br J Psychiatry 2013;203:288–96.
177. Willner P, Rose J, Jahoda A, et al. A cluster randomised controlled trial of a manualised cognitive behavioural anger management intervention delivered by supervised lay therapists to people with intellectual disabilities. Health Technol Assess 2013;17(21):1–173, v–vi.
178. Alpert JE, Spillmann MK. Psychotherapeutic approaches to aggressive and violent patients. Psychiatr Clin North Am 1997;20(2):453–72.
179. Teichner G, Golden CJ, Giannaris WJ. A multimodal approach to treatment of aggression in a severely brain-injured adolescent. Rehabil Nurs 1999;24(5): 207–11.
180. Alderman N, Davies JA, Jones C, et al. Reduction of severe aggressive behaviour in acquired brain injury: case studies illustrating clinical use of the OAS-MNR in the management of challenging behaviours. Brain Inj 1999; 13(9):669–704.
181. Pabis DJ, Stanislav SW. Pharmacotherapy of aggressive behavior. Ann Pharmacother 1996;30(3):278–87.
182. Hankin CS, Bronstone A, Koran LM. Agitation in the inpatient psychiatric setting: a review of clinical presentation, burden, and treatment. J Psychiatr Pract 2011; 17(3):170–85.
183. Allen MH, Currier GW, Carpenter D, et al. The expert consensus guideline series. Treatment of behavioral emergencies 2005. J Psychiatr Pract 2005; 11(Suppl 1):5–108 [quiz: 110–2].
184. Rao N, Jellinek HM, Woolston DC. Agitation in closed head injury: haloperidol effects on rehabilitation outcome. Arch Phys Med Rehabil 1985;66(1):30–4.
185. American Psychiatric Association. Quick reference to the American Psychiatric Association practice guidelines for the treatment of psychiatric disorders: compendium 2006. Arlington (VA): American Psychiatric Association; 2006.
186. Scott LK, Green R, McCarthy PJ, et al. Agitation and/or aggression after traumatic brain injury in the pediatric population treated with ziprasidone. Clinical article. J Neurosurg Pediatr 2009;3(6):484–7.
187. Michals ML, Crismon ML, Roberts S, et al. Clozapine response and adverse effects in nine brain-injured patients. J Clin Psychopharmacol 1993;13(3): 198–203.

Traumatic Brain Injury and Posttraumatic Stress Disorder

Nazanin H. Bahraini, PhD[a,b,*], Ryan E. Breshears, PhD[c,d],
Theresa D. Hernández, PhD[a,e], Alexandra L. Schneider, BA[a],
Jeri E. Forster, PhD[a,f], Lisa A. Brenner, PhD, ABPP[a,b,g,h]

KEYWORDS

- Brain injury • Posttraumatic stress • Imaging • Pathophysiology • Evaluation
- Treatment

KEY POINTS

- Individually, traumatic brain injury and posttraumatic stress disorder are complex conditions, and symptoms may be more difficult to address when the two co-occur.
- Evidence-based interventions aimed at treating both conditions simultaneously are limited; however, symptoms, regardless of cause, can be addressed by implementing treatment strategies aimed at ameliorating specific complaints (eg, headaches).
- Future research regarding the natural history of the co-occurring disorders can best be ascertained using longitudinal methodologies:
  - Cohorts with one, both, or neither of the conditions should be included;
  - Outcomes of interest should be measured via multiple modalities (eg, structured clinical interview, neuroimaging).

Disclaimer: this article is based on work supported, in part, by the Department of Veterans Affairs, but does not necessarily represent the views of the Department of Veterans Affairs or the United States government.

[a] Department of Veterans Affairs, Veteran Integrated Service Network (VISN) 19 Mental Illness Research Education and Clinical Center (MIRECC), 1055 Clermont Street, Denver, CO 80220, USA; [b] Department of Psychiatry, School of Medicine, University of Colorado, 13001 East 17th Place, Aurora, CO 80045, USA; [c] Wellstar Health System, Psychological Services, 55 Whitcher Street, Suite 420, Marietta, GA 30060, USA; [d] Department of Counseling and Human Development, University of Georgia, 402 Aderhold Hall, Athens, GA 30602, USA; [e] Department of Psychology and Neuroscience, University of Colorado, 1905 Colorado Avenue, Boulder, CO 80309, USA; [f] Department of Biostatistics & Informatics, Colorado School of Public Health, University of Colorado Denver, 13001 E. 17th Place, Aurora, CO 80045, USA; [g] Department of Neurology, School of Medicine, University of Colorado, 13001 E. 17th Place, Aurora, CO 80045, USA; [h] Department of Physical Medicine and Rehabilitation, School of Medicine, University of Colorado, 13001 E. 17th Place, Aurora, CO 80045, USA
* Corresponding author. Veteran Integrated Service Network (VISN) 19 Mental Illness Research Education and Clinical Center (MIRECC), 1055 Clermont Street, Denver, CO 80220.
E-mail address: nazanin.bahraini@va.gov

Psychiatr Clin N Am 37 (2014) 55–75
http://dx.doi.org/10.1016/j.psc.2013.11.002
0193-953X/14/$ – see front matter Published by Elsevier Inc.

psych.theclinics.com

Abbreviations	
PTSD	Posttraumatic stress disorder
TBI	Traumatic brain injury
mTBI	Mild traumatic brain injury
OEF/OIF/OND	Operation Enduring Freedom/Operation Iraqi Freedom/Operation New Dawn
LOC	Loss of consciousness
SCID	Structured Clinical Interview for DSM Disorders
CAPS	Clinician Administered PTSD Scale
PCL	PTSD Checklist
VHA	Veterans Heath Administration
vmPFC	Ventromedial prefrontal cortex
PTSS	Posttraumatic stress symptoms
SFG	Superior frontal gyrus
DTI	Diffusion tensor imaging
MDD	Major depressive disorder
FA	Fractional anisotropy
fMRI	Functional magnetic resonance imaging
OSU TBI-ID	Ohio State University TBI Identification
TSI	Trauma Symptom Inventory
VA	Departments of Veterans Affairs
DoD	Department of defense
CPG	Clinical practice guidelines
CT	Computed tomography
MOCA	Montreal Cognitive Assessment
SNRI	Serotonin norepinephrine reuptake inhibitor
CPT	Cognitive processing therapy
PE	Prolonged exposure

INTRODUCTION

It has been well established that traumatic brain injury (TBI) results in an increased risk for psychiatric illness, including mood and anxiety disorders, substance abuse, sleep disorders, and psychosis.[1–5] This situation is true even among individuals without a preexisting psychiatric history.[1–5] Although depression is the most prevalent psychiatric disorder observed in those with TBI,[4,6] anxiety disorders are also common and frequently coexist with depression. Studies have shown that individuals with TBI experience all variants of anxiety disorders, including generalized anxiety disorder, panic disorder, obsessive compulsive disorder, and posttraumatic stress disorder (PTSD).[1,3] However, in recent years, PTSD has been the most widely studied anxiety disorder in the context of TBI, particularly among those with mild TBI (mTBI).

The increased focus on PTSD and TBI has largely been motivated by the high rates of these conditions among Operation Enduring Freedom (OEF)/Operation Iraqi Freedom (OIF)/Operation New Dawn (OND) service members. Notwithstanding the greater historical context that has brought on heightened interest in this area, there are several reasons why the relationship between TBI and PTSD warrants special consideration. First, unlike other psychiatric disorders, PTSD is unique, in that its onset is tied to a discrete event, namely a psychologically traumatic stressor. Second, brain injuries resulting from biomechanical trauma are frequently sustained in the midst of psychologically traumatic experiences.[7] Similarities in the neuroanatomies of PTSD and TBI further suggest that the overlap in symptoms associated with both conditions may be the result of shared underlying mechanisms.[8]

Individually, TBI and PTSD are complex conditions, each of which can result in neurologic, cognitive, and behavioral symptoms. Symptom overlap and lack of objective and specific diagnostic aids or markers to facilitate rapid differential diagnosis make it difficult to separate the effects of TBI from those of PTSD. This situation is particularly true among those with mTBI. Differential diagnosis is even more challenging when there is a significant time lapse between the injury/stressor and formal evaluation. In light of these challenges, efforts are being refocused on increasing understanding regarding the complex interaction between biomechanically and psychologically traumatic events and their cumulative impact on neuropsychiatric outcomes.

Given the upsurge of PTSD and TBI research over the past decade, much of which has focused on those who have served in Iraq and Afghanistan, the purpose of this article is to review the literature published after September, 2001 (post–9/11 era) that addresses the co-occurrence of PTSD and TBI. This review begins with an overview of the epidemiology of co-occurring PTSD and TBI (all levels of injury severity). Second, neurobiological and neuropsychological correlates associated with both conditions are highlighted. Third, issues related to differential diagnosis and assessment of PTSD and TBI among individuals with both conditions are discussed. The current evidence regarding pharmacological and psychological treatments of PTSD and postconcussive symptoms in those with both TBI and PTSD are reviewed. Assessment and treatment considerations are also highlighted in a case vignette.

EPIDEMIOLOGY
Definitions of TBI and PTSD

TBI is defined as an alteration in brain function caused by an external force (ie, objects penetrating the brain, the head striking or being struck by an object, acceleration or deceleration of the brain, or exposure to forces associated with blasts).[9] Signs of alteration in brain function may include loss of consciousness (LOC), alteration in mental status, such as being dazed or confused, loss of memory for the event, or focal neurological deficits.[9] TBI can be further classified into 3 severity levels: mild, moderate, and severe.

Each year in the United States at least 1.7 million TBIs are sustained, most of which are of mild initial severity.[10,11] Individuals with a TBI may experience a range of symptoms after injury, including cognitive deficits in memory, attention, and concentration; physical or somatic complaints of fatigue, disordered sleep, dizziness, and headache; and affective complaints of irritability, anxiety, and depression. Many of these nonspecific symptoms are also associated with mental health conditions, such as PTSD and depression, which are frequent among those with TBI. Furthermore, the severity of TBI sequelae and the extent to which they persist are not linearly associated with injury severity.[12] Outcomes are dependent on a variety of psychological and contextual factors.[13]

PTSD is an anxiety disorder that results from exposure to a traumatic event that poses actual or threatened death or injury.[14] The diagnostic criteria for PTSD presented in the *Diagnostic and Statistical Manual of Mental Disorders, Fourth Edition Text Revision* (DSM-IV-TR)[15] required the individual to experience intense fear, helplessness, or horror in response to the traumatic event exposure, but this requirement was eliminated in the *Diagnostic and Statistical Manual of Mental Disorders, Fifth Edition* (DSM-5).[14] Another necessary component of PTSD diagnosis is the presence of specific trauma-related symptoms (DSM-5 criteria B–E), which must be present for at least a month (DSM-5 criterion F) and cause clinically significant distress or functional impairment (DSM-5 criterion G).[14] PTSD symptoms are grouped into

4 categories or clusters: reexperiencing of the traumatic event (eg, intrusive thoughts, nightmares); persistent symptoms of increased arousal (eg, hypervigilance, irritability); negative alterations in cognitions and mood associated with the traumatic events (eg, negative beliefs, expectations, and emotions, diminished interests, detachment); and avoidance of trauma-related stimuli (eg, thoughts, feelings, people, activities).[14]

The estimated lifetime prevalence of PTSD in the US general adult population using DSM-IV-TR criteria is approximately 8.7%.[14] However, substantially higher rates have been observed in subpopulations (eg, combat veterans).[16] Many of the population experience events that meet criteria for a PTSD stressor,[17] yet only a few individuals go on to develop PTSD. Moreover, research has shown that symptom severity and duration are affected by a multitude of factors, including characteristics of the traumatic stressor, preexisting history, and individual factors, as well as posttrauma variables (eg, social support).[18]

Frequency of PTSD Among TBI Survivors

Historically, the idea that PTSD and TBI can co-occur has been highly debated.[19] Although considerable work over the past decade has shown that PTSD and TBI, can and often do, coexist, findings from this and other reviews[20,21] raise questions regarding the prevalence of PTSD among those with TBI. As shown in **Fig. 1** (civilian samples) and **Fig. 2** (military samples), the frequencies of PTSD across levels of TBI severity vary substantially by population studied. Civilian estimates of PTSD range from 12% to 30% (mTBI), 15% to 27% (moderate TBI), and 3% to 23% (severe TBI).[1,6,22–34] Among military and veteran samples with TBI, estimates of PTSD range from 12% to 89%.[35–50] Differences in study purpose (eg, prevalence was primary

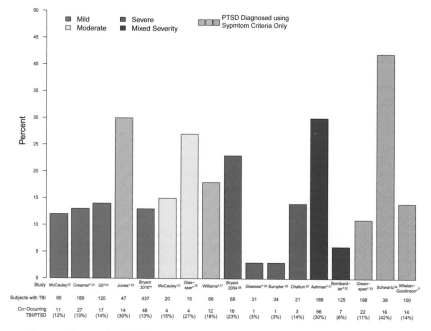

*Frequency of co-occurring TBI/PTSD as primary aim
All studies used clinical interview and/or medical record review to determine TBI status

Fig. 1. Frequency of co-occurring TBI and PTSD in studies with civilian populations.

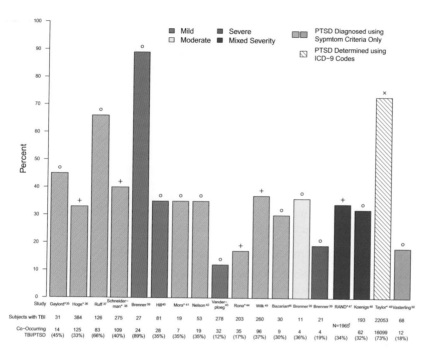

Fig. 2. Frequency of co-occurring TBI and PTSD in studies with Military/Veteran populations.

objective), sample size, subpopulations examined, case ascertainment of PTSD and TBI history, and methodologies used contribute to these variations.

With respect to PTSD case ascertainment, almost all of the civilian studies identified used diagnostic interviews, such as the Structured Clinical Interview for DSM Disorders[51] or the Clinician Administered PTSD Scale (CAPS)[52] to determine diagnosis. In contrast, military and veteran studies usually relied on symptom questionnaires, such as the PTSD Checklist (PCL).[53] This situation is potentially problematic, in that studies that use the PCL to estimate frequency of PTSD capture individuals that meet PTSD symptom criteria as opposed to full diagnostic criteria. Moreover, responses on symptom questionnaires may be influenced by a multitude of psychological and contextual factors (eg, motivational needs and comorbid conditions). Misattribution of symptoms to psychological trauma is also likely given the nonspecific nature of some PTSD symptoms. Taken together, these issues may contribute to an overestimation of PTSD when using symptom-based measures as the sole source of diagnosis in those with TBI. Several studies that compared frequencies of PTSD among those with TBI using different measures (self-report vs structured clinical interview) show that use of symptom-based self-report measures yield significantly higher estimates than structured interviews (59% vs 3%[29] and 33% vs 14%).[30–34]

As discussed in several previous publications (eg, Ref.[54]) significant challenges also exist in terms of determining history of TBI exposure, particularly when there is a significant time lapse between the injury/stressor and formal evaluation. TBI status for most of the military/veteran studies highlighted in **Fig. 2** was based on patient-administered

TBI screening measures. This situation is particularly problematic, because a recent study of the TBI screen within the Veterans Heath Administration reported that only about 55% of those with positive TBI screens subsequently had their injuries confirmed during a clinician-administered evaluation.[55] Even when a careful history is taken by a trained clinician, accurate diagnosis of TBI, particularly mTBI, is challenging, given its reliance on patient self-report. In a recent addition to this discussion, Xydakis and colleagues[56] investigated TBI identification and grading criteria with a specific emphasis on the role of LOC among a cohort of troops acutely injured during combat operations. Findings showed that among individuals with mTBI, those with self-reported LOC were significantly less likely than those without LOC to have abnormal neuroimaging. Although counterintuitive, these results, which have been found in other studies,[57,58] suggest that reported history of LOC should not automatically result in a definitive diagnosis of mTBI. Instead, LOC may be "more appropriately viewed as a neurophysiological response to trauma that may represent either a coincident indicator of whole-body trauma," or in other cases, a "potential maker for possible neurologic injury" (p.680).

The Influence of TBI on the Development and Course of PTSD

Several studies have reported that physical injury in the context of a psychologically traumatic event increases risk for PTSD.[59] There is also some evidence to suggest that compared with other bodily injuries, TBI confers additional risk of PTSD.[1,35–41,43–45] With respect to PTSD symptom severity, individuals with PTSD and mTBI endorse significantly more severe PTSD symptoms compared with those with PTSD alone.[60,61] Although research examining the longitudinal course of PTSD after TBI has been limited, some studies have found a reduction of symptoms over time,[1] whereas others have shown that TBI may complicate or prolong recovery from preexisting or comorbid conditions such as PTSD.[43] There is also some evidence that co-occurring PTSD and mTBI result in greater severity of postconcussive symptoms than either condition alone.[38,62] For example, in a cross-sectional study of injured OEF/OIF Soldiers from a Brigade Combat Team, Brenner and colleagues[62] showed that a combination of mTBI and PTSD was more strongly associated with a higher prevalence of each specific symptom, as well as any symptom, than either condition alone. In another study of Vietnam-era veterans, Vanderploeg and colleagues[43] found that mTBI and PTSD contributed independently to variance in a range of somatic, cognitive, and emotional symptoms. Taken together, these studies support the bidirectional relationship between mTBI and PTSD and their potential additive impact on signs and symptoms.

NEUROBIOLOGY OF CO-OCCURRING TBI AND PTSD

One of the most difficult challenges facing researchers interested in understanding the neural mechanisms underlying PTSD and TBI is the extraordinary variability of responses to both biomechanical and psychological trauma. Significant heterogeneity exists in terms of symptom expression across cohorts of individuals with TBI or PTSD. In part, this heterogeneity complicates identification of biomarkers for the diagnosis or prognosis of TBI or PTSD and limits current understanding regarding: (1) how history of TBI is associated with higher rates of PTSD among military personnel; and (2) why those with a history of TBI and co-occurring PTSD endorse more symptoms than those with either condition alone.

The collective evidence shows many overlapping deficits when PTSD and TBI are examined individually. (For review, see Brenner[63]; Simmons and Matthews[64]; Stein and McAllister[65]; Vasterling and colleagues[66]). However, there is a dearth of literature examining the underlying neural mechanisms and outcomes (eg, neuropsychological functioning[42,67]) when they co-occur. With respect to pathophysiology, some have proposed that the link between TBI and PTSD is merely incidental, because events that cause brain injury are frightening and may be more life-threatening than other injuries.[36] However, others have suggested that TBI and PTSD may be linked in a more instrumental way.[68] Many of the structural and neurochemical changes associated with TBI share similarities with pathophysiological change associated with PTSD.[69] For example, the pathogenesis of PTSD after trauma exposure has been conceptualized to involve a fear conditioning process in which fear responses are exaggerated or resistant to extinction.[70–72] Furthermore, the cause and maintenance of this fear conditioning have been hypothesized to involve multiple interacting neurobiological systems, including increased activation of the amygdala and reduced inhibitory control by the ventromedial prefrontal cortex (vmPFC) and the hippocampus.[73] Thus, damage to the frontal regions of the brain secondary to TBI may disrupt neural networks that play a prominent role in emotional regulation, making individuals more vulnerable to the effects of psychological trauma.[68] In this sense, TBI may introduce an additional liability, which when combined with other preexisting vulnerabilities (eg, genetic, environmental) may increase an individual's risk for developing PTSD.

Although there has been substantial discussion about the neural mechanisms underlying TBI and PTSD on a conceptual level, more research is needed to empirically characterize the complexity and direction of their interaction. Reger and colleagues[74] delineated the putative link between concussive injury and PTSD by combining 2 well-established and validated animal models: lateral fluid percussion injury (LFPI) (eg, concussion) and Pavlovian fear conditioning (eg, PTSD) to examine the impact of brain injury on neurobehavioral processes implicated in PTSD To test this theory, 48 hours after animals sustained LFPI, each was trained on fear conditioning, and then learned fear was assessed. Injured animals, compared with sham, showed both behavioral and molecular signs of enhanced reactivity of fear circuitry. Specifically, injured animals' learning was not impaired and was instead enhanced. In addition, their expression of fear was enhanced in relation to both the cue and the context. The molecular biomarker that corroborates this finding was the NR1 submit of the N-methyl-D-aspartate receptor in the basolateral amygdala complex, which was found to have increased 2 weeks after injury. These findings support the hypothesis that injury, like that sustained in a concussion, may result in alterations in neural circuitry and excitatory/inhibitory balance, which contribute to a lower threshold or enhanced responsively to fear-related stressors, thereby increasing the likelihood of developing PTSD. Still, data are emerging and remain equivocal, in that the impact of TBI on fear conditioning as a model of PTSD is not necessarily uniform and seems to be influenced by the type of injury model used.[75] Particularly in the case of mTBI, wherein the changes in fear conditioning are short-lived, more research is needed to understand the relevance of these findings to the pathophysiology of a chronic condition such as PTSD.

When trying to parse out the nature of individual contributions to co-occurring TBI/PTSD, animal models can be useful, because they allow for more control of potential variables. However, when these issues can be studied in humans with and without TBI and PTSD, this allows for an opportunity to take a reductionist view of what the key factors are as each contributes to the manifestation of symptoms associated with TBI and PTSD. To this end, there is some emerging evidence in humans suggesting that structural changes associated with TBI may increase risk for PTSD or subclinical posttraumatic stress symptoms.[76,77]

Imaging and Lesion-Behavioral Correlates

Rather than studying activation patterns or regional volume loss after the development of PTSD, Herskovits and colleagues[76] investigated the psychiatric effects of TBI by examining the impact of lesions induced by TBI on development of PTSD and individual PTSD symptom clusters 1 year after TBI in a sample of 97 children, adolescents, and young adults. Lesions in the right medial frontal and left middle temporal gyri were associated with PTSD diagnosis, such that lesion burden in the left middle temporal gyrus was positively associated with PTSD diagnosis, whereas an inverse association was found between lesion burden in the right medial frontal gyrus and a diagnosis of PTSD.

In another study, Max and colleagues[77] assessed the nature, rate, predictive factors, and neuroimaging correlates of novel (new-onset) definite and subclinical anxiety disorders 6 months after TBI. Novel definite/subclinical anxiety disorder: (1) was significantly and independently associated with lesions of the superior frontal gyrus (SFG) and novel definite/subclinical depressive disorder; and (2) showed a trend relationship with frontal white matter lesions. Furthermore, these findings could not be accounted for by differences in socioeconomic status, gender, race, preinjury psychiatric status, preinjury family functioning, severity of injury, or preinjury adaptive functioning. Although the outcome of interest included a heterogeneous group of anxiety disorders (PTSD, separation anxiety, generalized anxiety disorder, and panic disorder), definite and subclinical PTSD was the most prevalent anxiety disorder in the sample. This model implicates that dysfunction in the dorsal frontal neural system, including the SFG, may result in poor regulation of the affective states generated by the ventral neural system and may play a role in the onset of new anxiety symptoms after injury.

The studies highlighted earlier used prospective designs to examine the impact of TBI-related damage on subsequent development of PTSD or anxiety disorders. No prospective studies were identified that examined the impact of TBI-associated deficits on subsequent development of PTSD in adult populations. However, several recent cross-sectional studies in military samples may offer some additional insight into the potential impact of TBI on the development of PTSD. For example, data from a sample of Vietnam veterans with penetrating injuries showed that lesions involving the vmPFC and amygdala were significantly associated with a decreased prevalence of PTSD.[48–50] Furthermore, findings indicated that the reduced occurrence of PTSD associated with damage to these areas did not selectively diminish the frequency or intensity of individual categories of PTSD symptoms, but rather was the result of an overall reduction of symptoms across all 3 symptom categories.

In a study using diffusion tensor imaging (DTI), Matthews and colleagues[78] examined the effects of LOC, major depressive disorder (MDD), and PTSD on white matter integrity among individuals with combat-related mTBI and found that compared with those with alteration of consciousness (AOC), those with LOC showed significant disruption of white matter, as shown by lower fractional anisotropy in several regions in prefrontal cortex that are involved in the processing and regulation of emotion. Although there were no significant differences in white matter integrity between individuals with PTSD and those without PTSD (similar results were obtained in MDD vs non-MDD individuals), those with LOC compared with those with AOC had a higher prevalence of PTSD and MDD and more severe depressive and PTSD symptoms.[78] The investigators concluded that history of concussion with LOC was associated with detectable alterations in brain regions involved in emotional regulation and processing, which may increase risk of developing psychiatric symptoms after mTBI.[78]

Another study was performed using neuroimaging in 52 OEF/OIF combatants to parse out the contributions of and interactions among exposure to traumatic events and blasts, and history of TBI, as well as PTSD and TBI symptoms and the degree to which these individually or in combination could be accounted for by neuroanatomical markers in regions associated with PTSD.[46] The results showed that PTSD was not only associated with traumatic exposure during combat (including blast) but there was a significant correlation between neural abnormalities shown using DTI and PTSD severity. The investigators interpreted these findings to support the hypothesis that DTI changes may be more related to combat stress-related TBI, rather than the stress itself. Also of import was the finding of abnormal DTI in those with blast exposure, even without a report of mTBI.[46] The abnormalities shown with neuroimaging in those with PTSD and in those with exposure to blast need additional and more extensive characterization, in particular to determine if blast-related insult to brain tissue serves as a stepping stone for the development of PTSD.

Functional magnetic resonance imaging (fMRI), which indirectly measures brain activation during functional tasks, may be more sensitive to damage to neural networks caused by TBI.[79] For example, fMRI has been used to investigate many categories of neural processes and responses, such as working memory, emotional processing, and attention, as well as auditory and visual processing. In a recent review regarding the role of functional imaging to increase understanding regarding blast TBI, Graner and colleagues[79] highlighted the lack of existing fMRI research regarding mTBI and psychiatric comorbidities, particularly PTSD. Although no fMRI studies were identified that examined the interaction between PTSD and TBI, Simmons and Matthews[64] conducted 2 meta-analyses of published fMRI studies among PTSD or TBI populations in an attempt to quantitatively identify potential areas of overlap. Their findings showed the greatest overlap in the middle frontal gyrus; participants with PTSD showed more activation in this region compared with controls, whereas those with TBI showed hypoactivity. Although there were several methodological differences across studies, the investigators suggested that these findings may provide some insight into areas of significance for individuals who develop PTSD after TBI.

EVALUATION

Differential diagnosis, particularly in those with mTBI, can be challenging given the overlap in symptoms associated with TBI and PTSD, and the lack of objective markers for each condition. The evaluation process is complicated by patient-related characteristics (eg, poor recall of the event, premorbid conditions), or clinician-related factors (eg, confusion regarding cause, misattribution of symptom sequelae). For example, establishing whether the cause of altered consciousness experienced is biomechanical versus psychological can be impossible. Although TBI and PTSD are discrete conditions, with unique diagnostic criteria, accurate assessment may also be obscured by the provider's lack of understanding regarding diagnostic criteria. **Table 1** highlights the key diagnostic elements of each condition. With respect to cause, both TBI and PTSD are linked to a discrete event. However, the role of symptoms in diagnosing each condition is vastly different. Although the assessment of symptoms after TBI assists in identifying potential areas for intervention, TBI sequelae are neither necessary nor sufficient to establish a diagnosis of TBI. Rather, TBI is a historical event, and diagnosis is based on signs that occur at the time of an injury event (ie, external force resulting in an alteration of brain function). Thus, the presence or absence of postinjury symptoms is irrelevant to diagnosis.[54] Specifically, endorsement of symptoms after an

Table 1 Key diagnostic features of TBI and PTSD		
Criterion	TBI	PTSD[a]
Injury event/traumatic stressor	External force	Exposure to actual or threatened death, injury, or sexual violence to self or others (A)
Immediate response	Alteration of brain function	Not required
Symptoms	Not required	Intrusion, avoidance, negative alterations in cognition and mood, and hyperarousal (B–E)
Duration of symptoms	Not required	>30 d (F)
Functioning	Not required	Clinically significant impairment in key areas of functioning (G)

[a] Based on DSM-5 criteria.
Data from American Psychiatric Association. Diagnostic and statistical manual of mental disorders. 5th edition. Arlington (VA): American Psychiatric Association; 2013. Available at: dsm.psychiatryonline.org. Accessed November 5, 2013.

injury, such as headaches, memory problems, fatigue, and irritability, does not confirm that the individual sustained a TBI. Moreover, not having current symptoms does not mean that the person did not sustain a TBI. Most individuals who sustain mTBIs or concussions recover fully within weeks after injury without any residual symptoms. Symptom endorsement may be related to the TBI but may also be associated with other factors or co-occurring conditions. Conversely, current symptom endorsement after trauma exposure (eg, reexperiencing of the traumatic event, avoidance of trauma-related stimuli, and hyperarousal) is a necessary component of PTSD diagnosis.[14]

In light of the challenges noted earlier, careful assessment of both conditions using valid and reliable instruments is essential. Although hospital records or neuroimaging findings may assist with the historical diagnosis of more severe or acute injury, the gold standard for determining previous TBI, particularly mTBI and PTSD, is a face-to-face clinical interview by a health professional who has received training regarding diagnostic criteria. This method is often cited as the gold standard by which the diagnostic usefulness of other measures is evaluated. There is no commonly used screening, assessment, or diagnostic tool tailored to evaluate history or sequelae of comorbid mTBI and PTSD or to assist in differential diagnosis. However, assessment of each condition individually can be enhanced by using psychometrically sound structured clinical interview measures, such as the Ohio State University TBI Identification[80] for TBI and the CAPS[52] for PTSD.

As discussed earlier, self-report measures of signs and symptoms should not be used as stand-alone tools for diagnostic purposes, because they have limited usefulness in terms of differential diagnosis and may contribute to symptom misattribution. When used in conjunction with diagnostic interviews or other clinician-administered assessments, self-report measures of symptoms may offer providers some insight into areas that patients perceive as most problematic. However, attribution of symptoms to a specific condition or cause may not be possible.[81] For example, in a recent psychometric study of the Neurobehavioral Symptom Inventory (NSI),[82] a self-report measure of postconcussive symptoms, OEF/OIF veterans with PTSD only or depression only had significantly higher NSI scores than those with TBI only.[83] Furthermore, total NSI scores linearly increased with the number of conditions met, such that individuals with all 4 conditions examined (ie, TBI, PTSD, depression, and generalized anxiety) scored higher than those with 2 or 3 of these conditions.[83] Such findings highlight the significant limitations of existing self-report measures commonly used to assess postconcussive symptoms in those with a history of TBI, and their inability to differentiate true postconcussive symptoms from affective and cognitive symptoms occurring in the context of psychiatric illness. In addition, few studies have evaluated the psychometric properties of commonly used self-report measures of PTSD symptoms in TBI populations. Bahraini and colleagues[84] suggested that the Trauma Symptom Inventory[85] is a useful measure of PTSD symptoms in those who may also have a TBI, including those with mTBI.

Neuroimaging and Neuropsychological Assessment

Although there is evidence of neuropsychological deficits that may be unique to the co-occurrence of mTBI and PTSD (eg, processing speed and executive functioning),[42,67] no neuropsychological assessment or profile is associated with PTSD, TBI, or their comorbidity that can aid in differential diagnosis of individual patients.[86] Research does indicate that neuropsychological test results may aid in the identification of cognitive impairment after mTBI, particularly during the acute phase. Immediately after injury, neuropsychological results may be more effective than subjective reports of symptoms in differentiating between injured and noninjured individuals.[87] However, in the chronic phase, the diagnostic (injured vs noninjured) usefulness of these measures is limited. Nevertheless, neuropsychological assessment can be used in conjunction with other forms of evaluation to determine level of impairment, identify consequences of illness or injury, or evaluate changes in functioning.

With respect to imaging, methods often used in clinical practice are not sensitive to all TBIs (eg, less severe injury, injuries sustained many years previously [childhood injuries]).[87] The frequent lack of objective findings restricts the usefulness of these procedures.[87] According to the Departments of Veterans Affairs (VA) and Defense (DoD) clinical practice guidelines (CPG) for mTBI,[88] computed tomography (CT) scan is the modality of choice as a diagnostic tool for acute concussion/mTBI. However, the absence of abnormal findings on CT does not preclude the presence of concussion/mTBI. More advanced magnetic resonance imaging techniques, such as DTI, have shown promise in detecting changes associated with mTBI,[89] but additional research is needed to better understand their clinical usefulness.[90]

TREATMENT IMPLICATIONS

Without clear guidance regarding the simultaneous management of TBI and PTSD, working with patients to ameliorate symptoms associated with the conditions remains challenging. As shown in **Table 2**, research on pharmacological and psychological interventions for individuals with co-occurring TBI and PTSD is limited.[91–95] Although findings from these few studies are promising, most were uncontrolled trials that were conducted with small sample sizes. The effectiveness of current evidence-based treatments for PTSD or PTSD symptoms, such as cognitive processing therapy (CPT), prolonged exposure (PE), and prazosin for nightmares, have yet to be substantiated in those with co-occurring TBI. Given the limited amount of research, treatment of those with TBI and PTSD should involve a combination of psychoeducation, symptom management, and evidence-based treatments for PTSD and other comorbid behavioral health conditions. Psychoeducation is an important component of any intervention, particularly when delivered early after injury/trauma. VA/DoD CPG for both PTSD[96] and mTBI[88] emphasize the importance of educating patients to help normalize reactions, enhance self-care, and promote expectations for recovery.

Table 2
Pharmacological and psychotherapeutic intervention studies of TBI and PTSD

Source	Design	Sample/Setting	Intervention	Primary Outcome	Secondary Outcome(s)	Findings
Ruff et al,[91] 2009	Before-after	74 OEF/OIF veterans with mTBI (96% with PTSD) VA polytrauma clinic	Prazosin	Sleep (ESS)	HA pain and frequency Cognition (MOCA)	ESS (Δpre-post) 8.82; $P<.001$ HA pain (Δpre-post) 3.2; $P<.001$ HA frequency (Δpre-post) 7.63; $P<.001$ Cognition (Δpre-post) 4.1; $P<.001$
Chard et al,[92] 2011	Before-after	42 veterans with TBI (mild-severe) and PTSD Residential treatment program	CPT-C (group and individual sessions over 7 wk) Psychoeducation groups and cognitive rehabilitation	PTSD symptoms (CAPS total)	Depressive symptoms (BDI-II total)	PTSD sxs $P<.01$; $\eta^2 = .79$[a] Depressive sxs $P<.001$; $\eta^2 = .52$[a]
Walter et al,[93] 2012	Before-after	28 veterans with TBI (mild-moderate) and PTSD Residential treatment program	CPT-C (group and individual sessions over 8 wk) Psychoeducation groups and cognitive rehabilitation	PTSD symptoms (CAPS total)	PCS (NSI total)	PTSD sxs $P = .000$; $d = 1.43$[b] PCS $P = .001$; $d = .68$[b]
Wolf et al,[94] 2012	Before-after	10 OEF/OIF veterans with TBI (mild-moderate) and chronic PTSD Outpatient mental health/PTSD clinic	Prolonged exposure	PTSD symptoms (PCL)	Depressive symptoms (BDI-II total)	PTSD sxs $P<.001$; $d = 3.64$[b] Depressive sxs $P<.001$; $d = 1.82$[b]
Bryant et al,[95] 2003	RCT	24 civilian patients with mTBI and acute stress disorder Outpatient mental health clinic	CBT (5 weekly individual sessions) Control-supportive counseling	PTSD diagnosis (CAPS) after treatment	Anxiety (BAI total) Depressive symptoms (BDI-II total)	PTSD diagnosis CBT N = 1 (8%) Control N = 7 (58%) $P<.05$; $d = 1.16$[b]

Abbreviations: BAI, Beck Anxiety Inventory; BDI-II, Beck Depression Inventory-II; CBT, cognitive behavioral therapy; CPT-C, cognitive processing therapy cognitive-only; ESS, Epworth Sleepiness Scale; HA, headache; MOCA, Montreal Cognitive Assessment; PCS, postconcussive symptoms; RCT, randomized controlled trial; sxs, symptoms.
[a] η^2 effect size.
[b] effect size.

Moreover, providing early education to patients and their families is the best available treatment of preventing and reducing the development of persistent symptoms after mTBI.[97]

Symptom Management

In the face of diagnostic challenges, clinicians should be encouraged to identify and address symptoms, regardless of cause, in a stepwise fashion.[54] This practice is consistent with mTBI CPG recently published by the VA and DoD.[88] Similarly, treatment recommendations from the recently updated VA/DoD CPG for Management of Post-Traumatic Stress[96] are considered from the perspective of simultaneously managing comorbid TBI. When identifying treatment targets, consideration should be given to those that cut across both conditions and contribute to the greatest amount of patient distress and impairment in functioning. Chronic pain and sleep disturbance are common among individuals with TBI and PTSD, and improvements in these areas may contribute to reduction or even resolution of other symptoms.

In cases in which reexperiencing symptoms are contributing to sleep problems, there is some evidence to suggest that the α-blocker prazosin may mitigate the recurring nightmares and flashbacks that some PTSD sufferers report.[98–100] This is a particularly relevant consideration given: (1) the high prevalence of sleep disturbances reported among patients with PTSD[101]; and (2) that many of the more often used pharmacological aids to treat PTSD are associated with sleep interference. Although more research is needed, prazosin seems to be a promising treatment of sleep and headaches in veterans with a history of mTBI and co-occurring PTSD. Ruff and colleagues[91] conducted a before-after trial of prazosin to improve sleep and reduce headaches in a sample of 74 OEF/OIF veterans with a history of mTBI and residual neurocognitive deficits, of whom 71 had co-occurring PTSD. Results showed that prazosin was well tolerated, with a low incidence of side effects. Although this was not a controlled trial, those taking prazosin reported improved sleep, reduced daytime sleepiness, fewer headaches, less severe headache pain, and improved cognitive performance on the Montreal Cognitive Assessment (MOCA).[91] Given its recommended use for nightmares in PTSD, and the preliminary results of this open-label trial in those with mTBI, prazosin may be considered in veterans with both PTSD and TBI, but with a low starting dose and a slow upward titration to avoid hypotension.[97]

Pharmacological Treatments for PTSD and TBI

Although pharmacotherapy treatments are challenging with respect to either PTSD or TBI alone, the complexity of these conditions when co-occurring is substantial. Given that both PTSD and TBI are vulnerable to changes in a patient's environment, McAllister[81] recommended psychotropic trials at therapeutic dosing of no less than 2 weeks and emphasized the benefits of longer durations (4–8 weeks) when treatment is tolerated. With respect to specific drug classes that have been recommended individually for both conditions, selective serotonin reuptake inhibitor antidepressants sertraline and paroxetine and the serotonin norepinephrine reuptake inhibitor antidepressant venlafaxine are first-line medication choices for treating PTSD.[96] Findings also support use of sertraline as a first-line therapy for treating mood and anxiety disorders after TBI.[102]

Ascertaining pharmacological options from an arousal model may be useful, but they are also associated with risk of symptom exacerbation, representing a unique conundrum for treating TBI-PTSD co-occurrences. A patient with TBI, for example, may report symptoms of underarousal (eg, apathy), which could be mitigated with psychostimulant medications (eg, methylphenidate), but with the possibility of increasing the overarousal symptoms that often characterize PTSD.[81,97] Paradoxically, pharmacotherapy aimed at treating the overarousal symptoms of PTSD via an anxiolytic could result in the iatrogenic effect of exacerbating cognitive slowing and problems with memory and inattention (issues that are already inherent in the sequelae reported by many patients with TBI).

Psychotherapy for PTSD and TBI

Three studies were identified that examined the effect of evidence-based treatments for PTSD in those with a history of TBI. Chard and colleagues[92] found that a 7-week inpatient program consisting of CPT combined with cognitive rehabilitation and psychoeducation groups contributed to significant reductions in PTSD symptom scores among veterans with both TBI and PTSD. Furthermore, the reductions in PTSD symptoms were observed across all levels of TBI severity. In a more recent study, veterans in an 8-week residential PTSD/TBI program reported significant decreases in PTSD and postconcussive symptoms over the course of treatment.[93] The decrease in PTSD symptoms was significantly and positively associated with PC symptoms. In addition, a preliminary study of PE in veterans with comorbid TBI (mild to moderate) and PTSD[94] showed significant reductions in PTSD and depressive symptoms. Standard implementation of the PE manual was used in all cases, with slight adjustments to account for veterans' residual cognitive deficits (eg, electronic calendars, smart phones, increased structure).[94] Taken together, these findings are promising and suggest that evidence-based treatments for PTSD, with some minor modifications, may also be effective for those with a history of TBI.

Combined Interventions for PTSD and TBI

Although no studies were identified that investigated combined pharmacological and behavioral interventions exclusively in those with co-occurring TBI and PTSD, findings from a recent study conducted with 207 surgically hospitalized injury survivors (38% with mild to moderate TBI) using a stepped care approach may have important implications for individuals with TBI and PTSD.[103] Specifically, individuals who screened high for PSTD symptoms were randomized to a stepped combined care management, psychopharmacology, and cognitive behavioral psychotherapy intervention or usual care. Results, which were not reported separately for individuals with TBI, showed that over the course of the year after injury, those receiving the stepped care intervention had clinically significantly reduced PTSD symptoms at 6, 9, and 12 months after injury, as well as significant improvements in physical function.[103] In light of these findings, the investigators discussed the potential usefulness of introducing screening and intervention procedures for PTSD prevention in trauma centers.

SUMMARY

Although the literature on PTSD and TBI as individual conditions is vast, studies that address both PTSD and TBI as co-occurring conditions are limited. TBI and PTSD are individually complex and when combined may be mutually exacerbating. This situation creates significant assessment and treatment challenges. Nevertheless, emerging evidence highlighting neurobiological changes associated with TBI, which may be linked to the pathophysiology associated with PTSD, are promising and warrant more attention. In this vein, prospective studies that combine neuroimaging, neuropsychological assessment, and reliable and valid diagnostic measures of both TBI and PTSD are essential in clarifying how history of TBI is associated with a greater risk of developing PTSD, as well as why those with both conditions endorse more symptoms than those with either PTSD or TBI alone. Incorporating more advanced imaging techniques such as DTI or fMRI, especially in the case of mTBI and PTSD, is an important future direction. In terms of treatment, more studies are needed to examine the efficacy of psychopharmacological and behavioral interventions for various treatment targets among those with co-occurring TBI and PTSD. Along these lines, research focused on early intervention for specific risk factors (eg, acute stress symptoms/disorder) may be critical in preventing PTSD after trauma exposure in those who have sustained a TBI. Stepwise treatment of symptoms also seems promising. Future research should continue to be directed at studies of the comorbid state to fully characterize its relationship and impact on neuropsychiatric outcomes.

REFERENCES

1. Bryant RA, O'Donnell ML, Creamer M, et al. The psychiatric sequelae of traumatic injury. Am J Psychiatry 2010;167(3):312–20.
2. Fann JR, Burington B, Leonetti A, et al. Psychiatric illness following traumatic brain injury in an adult health maintenance organization population. Arch Gen Psychiatry 2004;61(1):53–61.
3. Hibbard MR, Uysal S, Kepler K, et al. Axis I psychopathology in individuals with traumatic brain injury. J Head Trauma Rehabil 1998;13(4):24–39.
4. Koponen S, Taiminen T, Portin R, et al. Axis I and II psychiatric disorders after traumatic brain injury: a 30-year follow-up study. Am J Psychiatry 2002;159(8): 1315–21.
5. Wei W, Sambamoorthi U, Crystal S, et al. Mental illness, traumatic brain injury, and Medicaid expenditures. Arch Phys Med Rehabil 2005;86(5):905–11.
6. Whelan-Goodinson R, Ponsford J, Johnston L, et al. Psychiatric disorders following traumatic brain injury: their nature and frequency. J Head Trauma Rehabil 2009;24(5):324–32.
7. Bryant R. Post-traumatic stress disorder vs traumatic brain injury. Dialogues Clin Neurosci 2011;13(3):251–62.
8. McAllister TW, Stein MB. Effects of psychological and biomechanical trauma on brain and behavior. Ann N Y Acad Sci 2010;1208:46–57.
9. Menon DK, Schwab K, Wright DW, et al. Position statement: definition of traumatic brain injury. Arch Phys Med Rehabil 2010;91(11):1637–40.
10. Centers for Disease Control and Prevention (CDC), National Center for Injury Prevention and Control. Report to Congress on mild traumatic brain injury in the United States: steps to prevent a serious public health problem. Atlanta (GA): Centers for Disease Control and Prevention; 2003.
11. Faul M, Xu L, Wald MM, et al. Traumatic brain injury in the United States:emergency department visits, hospitalizations, and deaths. Atlanta (GA): Centers for Disease Control and Prevention, National Center for Injury Prevention and Control; 2010.
12. Saltapidas H, Ponsford J. The influence of cultural background on motivation for and participation in rehabilitation and outcome following traumatic brain injury. J Head Trauma Rehabil 2007;22(2):132–9.
13. Whittaker R, Kemp S, House A. Illness perceptions and outcome in mild head injury: a longitudinal study. J Neurol Neurosurg Psychiatr 2007;78:644–6.
14. American Psychiatric Association. Diagnostic and statistical manual of mental disorders. 5th edition. Arlington (VA): American Psychiatric Association; 2013. Available at: dsm.psychiatryonline.org/. Accessed November 5, 2013.

15. American Psychiatric Association. Diagnostic and statistical manual of mental disorders. 4th edition text revision. Washington, DC: American Psychiatric Association; 2000.

16. Schlenger WE, Kulka R, Fairbank JA, et al. The prevalence of post-traumatic stress disorder in the Vietnam generation: a multimethod, multisource assessment of psychiatric disorder. J Trauma Stress 1992;5:333–63.

17. Breslau N, Kessler RC. The stressor criterion in SDM-IV posttraumatic stress disorder: an empirical investigation. Biol Psychiatry 2001;50(9):699–704.

18. Brewin CR, Andrews B, Valentine JD. Meta-analysis of risk factors for posttraumatic stress disorder in trauma-exposed adults. J Consult Clin Psychol 2000; 68(5):748–66.

19. Harvey AG, Brewin CR, Jones C, et al. Coexistence of posttraumatic stress disorder and traumatic brain injury: towards a resolution of the paradox. J Int Neuropsychol Soc 2003;9(4):663–76.

20. Carlson KF, Kehle SM, Meis LA, et al. Prevalence, assessment, and treatment of mild traumatic brain injury and posttraumatic stress disorder: a systematic review. J Head Trauma Rehabil 2011;26(2):103–15.

21. Ramchand R, Schell TL, Karney BR, et al. Disparate prevalence estimates of PTSD among service members who served in Iraq and Afghanistan: possible explanations. J Trauma Stress 2010;23(1):59–68.

22. McCauley SR, Boake C, Levin HS, et al. Postconcussional disorder following mild to moderate traumatic brain injury: anxiety, depression, and social support as risk factors and comorbidities. J Clin Exp Neuropsychol 2001;23(6):792–808.

23. Creamer M, O'Donnell ML, Pattison P. Amnesia, traumatic brain injury, and posttraumatic stress disorder: a methodological inquiry. Behav Res Ther 2005; 43(10):1383–9.

24. Gil S, Caspi Y, Ben-Ari IZ, et al. Does memory of a traumatic event increase the risk for posttraumatic stress disorder in patients with traumatic brain injury? A prospective study. Am J Psychiatry 2005;162(5):963–9.

25. Jones C, Harvey AG, Brewin CR. Traumatic brain injury, dissociation, and posttraumatic stress disorder in road traffic accident survivors. J Trauma Stress 2005;18(3):181–91.

26. Glaesser J, Neuner F, Lütgehetmann R, et al. Posttraumatic stress disorder in patients with traumatic brain injury. BMC Psychiatry 2004;4:5.

27. Williams WH, Evans JJ, Wilson BA, et al. Brief report: prevalence of posttraumatic stress disorder symptoms after severe traumatic brain injury in a representative community sample. Brain Inj 2002;16(8):673–9.

28. Bryant RA, Marosszeky JE, Crooks J, et al. Elevated resting heart rate as a predictor of posttraumatic stress disorder after severe traumatic brain injury. Psychosom Med 2004;66(5):760–1.

29. Sumpter RE, McMillan TM. Misdiagnosis of post-traumatic stress disorder following severe traumatic brain injury. Br J Psychiatry 2005;186:423–6.

30. Chalton LD, McMillian TM. Can 'partial' PTSD explain difference in diagnosis of PTSD by questionnaire self-report and interview after head injury? Brain Inj 2009;23(2):77–82.

31. Ashman TA, Spielman LA, Hibbard MR, et al. Psychiatric challenges in the first 6 years after traumatic brain injury: cross-sequential analyses of Axis I disorders. Arch Phys Med Rehabil 2004;85(4 Suppl 2):S36–42.

32. Bombardier CH, Fann JR, Temkin N, et al. Posttraumatic stress disorder symptoms during the first six months after traumatic brain injury. J Neuropsychiatry Clin Neurosci 2006;18(4):501–8.

33. Greenspan AI, Stringer AY, Phillips VL, et al. Symptoms of post-traumatic stress: intrusion and avoidance 6 and 12 months after TBI. Brain Inj 2006; 20(7):733–42.
34. Schwartz I, Tsenter J, Shochina M, et al. Rehabilitation outcomes of terror victims with multiple traumas. Arch Phys Med Rehabil 2007;88(4):440–8.
35. Gaylord KM, Cooper DB, Mercado JM, et al. Incidence of posttraumatic stress disorder and mild traumatic brain injury in burned service members: preliminary report. J Trauma 2008;64(Suppl 2):S200–6.
36. Hoge CW, McGurk D, Thomas JL, et al. Mild traumatic brain injury in U.S. soldiers returning from Iraq. N Engl J Med 2008;358(5):453–63.
37. Ruff RL, Ruff SS, Wang XF. Headaches among Operation Iraqi Freedom/Operation Enduring Freedom veterans with mild traumatic brain injury associated with exposures to explosions. J Rehabil Res Dev 2008;46:941–52.
38. Schneiderman AI, Braver ER, Kang HK. Understanding sequelae of injury mechanisms and mild traumatic brain injury incurred during the conflicts in Iraq and Afghanistan: persistent postconcussive symptoms and posttraumatic stress disorder. Am J Epidemiol 2008;167(12):1446–52.
39. Brenner LA, Ladley-O'Brien SE, Harwood JE, et al. An exploratory study of neuroimaging, neurologic, and neuropsychological findings in veterans with traumatic brain injury and/or posttraumatic stress disorder. Mil Med 2009;174(4): 347–52.
40. Hill JJ, Mobo BH, Cullen MR. Separating deployment-related traumatic brain injury and posttraumatic stress disorder in veterans: preliminary findings from the Veterans Affairs traumatic brain injury screening program. Am J Phys Med Rehabil 2009;88(8):605–14.
41. Mora AG, Ritenour AE, Wade CE, et al. Posttraumatic stress disorder in combat casualties with burns sustaining primary blast and concussive injuries. J Trauma 2009;66(Suppl 4):S178–85.
42. Nelson IA, Yoash-Gantz RE, Rickett TC, et al. Relationship between processing speed and executive functioning performance among OEF/OIF veterans: implications for postdeployment rehabilitation. J Head Trauma Rehabil 2009;24(1): 32–40.
43. Vanderploeg RD, Belanger HG, Curtiss G. Mild traumatic brain injury and posttraumatic stress disorder and their associations with health symptoms. Arch Phys Med Rehabil 2009;90(7):1084–93.
44. Rona RJ, Jones M, Fear NT, et al. Mild traumatic brain injury in UK military personnel returning from Afghanistan and Iraq: cohort and cross-sectional analyses. J Head Trauma Rehabil 2012;27(1):33–44.
45. Wilk JE, Herrell RK, Wynn GH, et al. Mild traumatic brain injury (concussion), posttraumatic stress disorder, and depression in U.S. soldiers involved in combat deployments: association with postdeployment symptoms. Psychosom Med 2012;74(3):249–57.
46. Bazarian JJ, Donnelly K, Peterson DR, et al. The relation between posttraumatic stress disorder and mild traumatic brain injury acquired during Operations Enduring Freedom and Iraqi Freedom. J Head Trauma Rehabil 2013;28(1):1–12.
47. RAND Center for Military Health Policy Research. Invisible wounds of war: psychological and cognitive injuries, their consequences, and services to assist recovery. Santa Monica (CA): RAND; 2008.
48. Koenigs M, Huey ED, Raymont V, et al. Focal brain damage protects against post-traumatic stress disorder in combat veterans. Nat Neurosci 2008;11(2): 232–7.

49. Taylor BC, Hagel EM, Carlson KF, et al. Prevalence and costs of co-occurring traumatic brain injury with and without psychiatric disturbance and pain among Afghanistan and Iraq war veteran V.A. users. Med Care 2012;50(4):342–6.
50. Vasterling JJ, Brailey K, Proctor SP, et al. Neuropsychological outcomes of mild traumatic brain injury, post-traumatic stress disorder and depression in Iraqdeployed US Army soldiers. Br J Psychiatry 2012;201(3):186–92.
51. First MB, Spitzer RL, Gibbon M, et al. Structured clinical interview for DSM-IV-TR Axis I disorders. New York: Biometrics Research, New York State Psychiatric Institute; 2002.
52. Blake DD, Weathers FW, Nagy LM, et al. The development of a clinician administered PTSD scale. J Trauma Stress 1995;8(1):75–90.
53. Weathers F, Litz B, Herman D, et al. The PTSD Checklist (PCL): reliability, validity, and diagnostic utility. Presented at the Annual Meeting of the International Society for Traumatic Stress Studies. San Antonio, October, 1993.
54. Brenner LA, Vanderploeg RD, Terrio H. Assessment and diagnosis of mild traumatic brain injury, posttraumatic stress disorder, and other polytrauma conditions: burden of adversity hypothesis. Rehabil Psychol 2009;54(3):239–46.
55. Scholten JD, Sayer NA, Vanderploeg RD, et al. Analysis of US Veterans Health Administration comprehensive evaluations for traumatic brain injury in Operation Enduring Freedom and Operation Iraqi Freedom Veterans. Brain Inj 2012; 26(10):1177–84.
56. Xydakis MS, Ling GS, Mulligan LP, et al. Epidemiologic aspects of traumatic brain injury in acute combat casualties at a major military medical center: a cohort study. Ann Neurol 2012;72(5):673–81.
57. Haydel MJ, Shembekar AD. Prediction of intracranial injury in children aged five years and older with loss of consciousness after minor head injury due to nontrivial mechanisms. Ann Emerg Med 2003;42(4):507–14.
58. Palchak MJ, Holmes JF, Vance CW, et al. Does an isolated history of loss of consciousness or amnesia predict brain injuries in children after blunt head trauma? Pediatrics 2004;113(6):e507–13.
59. Koren D, Norman D, Cohen A, et al. Increased PTSD risk with combat-related injury: a matched comparison study of injured and uninjured soldiers experiencing the same combat events. Am J Psychiatry 2005;162:276–82.
60. Barnes SM, Walter KH, Chard KM. Does a history of mild traumatic brain injury increase suicide risk in veterans with PTSD? Rehabil Psychol 2012;57(1):18–26.
61. Ragsdale KA, Neer SM, Beidel DC, et al. Posttraumatic stress disorder in OEF/OIF veterans with and without traumatic brain injury. J Anxiety Disord 2013; 27(4):420–6.
62. Brenner LA, Ivins BJ, Schwab K, et al. Traumatic brain injury, posttraumatic stress disorder, and postconcussive symptom reporting among troops returning from Iraq. J Head Trauma Rehabil 2010;25(5):307–12.
63. Brenner LA. Neuropsychological and neuroimaging findings in traumatic brain injury and post-traumatic stress disorder. Dialogues Clin Neurosci 2011;13(3): 311–23.
64. Simmons AN, Matthews SC. Neural circuitry of PTSD with or without mild traumatic brain injury: a meta-analysis. Neuropharmacology 2012;62(2):598–606.
65. Stein MB, McAllister TW. Exploring the convergence of posttraumatic stress disorder and mild traumatic brain injury. Am J Psychiatry 2009;166(7):768–76.
66. Vasterling JJ, Verfaellie M, Sullivan KD. Mild traumatic brain injury and posttraumatic stress disorder in returning veterans: perspectives from cognitive neuroscience. Clin Psychol Rev 2009;29(8):674–84.

67. Campbell TA, Nelson LA, Lumpkin R. Neuropsychological measures of processing speed and executive functioning in combat veterans with PTSD, TBI, and comorbid TBI/PTSD. Psychiatr Ann 2009;39(8):796–803.
68. Bryant R. Disentangling mild traumatic brain injury and stress reactions. N Engl J Med 2008;358:525–7.
69. Kennedy JE, Jaffee MS, Leskin GA, et al. Posttraumatic stress disorder and posttraumatic stress disorder-like symptoms and mild traumatic brain injury. J Rehabil Res Dev 2007;44(7):895–920.
70. Keane TM, Scott WO, Chavoya GA, et al. Social support in Vietnam veterans with posttraumatic stress disorder: a comparative analysis. J Consult Clin Psychol 1985;53(1):95–102.
71. Amstadter AB, Nugent NR, Koenen KC, et al. Association between COMT, PTSD, and increased smoking following hurricane exposure in an epidemiologic sample. Psychiatry 2009;72(4):360–9.
72. Jovanovic T, Ressler KJ. How the neurocircuitry and genetics of fear inhibition may inform our understanding of PTSD. Am J Psychiatry 2010;167(6):648–62.
73. Milad MR, Pitman RK, Ellis CB, et al. Neurobiological basis of failure to recall extinction memory in posttraumatic stress disorder. Biol Psychiatry 2009; 66(12):1075–82.
74. Reger ML, Poulos AM, Buen F, et al. Concussive brain injury enhances fear learning and excitatory processes in the amygdala. Biol Psychiatry 2012; 71(4):335–43.
75. Genovese RF, Simmons LP, Ahlers ST, et al. Effects of mild TBI from repeated blast overpressure on the expression and extinction of conditioned fear in rats. Neuroscience 2013;254:120–9.
76. Herskovits EH, Gerring JP, Davatzikos C, et al. Is the spatial distribution of brain lesions associated with closed-head injury in children predictive of subsequent development of posttraumatic stress disorder? Radiology 2002;224(2): 345–51.
77. Max JE, Keatley E, Wilde EA, et al. Anxiety disorders in children and adolescents in the first six months after traumatic brain injury. J Neuropsychiatry Clin Neurosci 2011;23(1):29–39.
78. Matthews SC, Spadoni AD, Lohr JB, et al. Diffusion tensor imaging evidence of white matter disruption associated with loss versus alteration of consciousness in warfighters exposed to combat in Operations Enduring and Iraqi Freedom. Psychiatry Res 2012;204(2–3):149–54.
79. Graner J, Oakes TR, French LM, et al. Functional MRI in the investigation of blast-related traumatic brain injury. Front Neurol 2012;4:16.
80. Corrigan JD, Bogner J. Initial reliability and validity of the Ohio State University TBI identification. J Head Trauma Rehabil 2007;22(6):318–29.
81. McAllister TW. Psychopharmacological issues in the treatment of TBI and PTSD. Clin Neuropsychol 2009;23(8):1338–67.
82. Cicerone KD, Kalmar K. Persistent postconcussion syndrome: the structure of subjective complaints after mild traumatic brain injury. J Head Trauma Rehabil 1995;10(3):1–17.
83. King PR, Donnelly KT, Donnelly JP, et al. Psychometric study of the Neurobehavioral Symptom Inventory. J Rehabil Res Dev 2012;49(6):879–88.
84. Bahraini NH, Brenner LA, Harwood JE, et al. Utility of the trauma symptom inventory for the assessment of post-traumatic stress symptoms in veterans with a history of psychological trauma and/or brain injury. Mil Med 2009;174(10): 1005–9.

85. Briere J. Trauma symptom inventory professional manual. Odessa (FL): Psychological Assessment Resources; 1995.
86. Dolan S, Martindale S, Robinson J, et al. Neuropsychological sequelae of PTSD and TBI following war deployment among OEF/OIF veterans. Neuropsychol Rev 2012;22(1):21–34.
87. McCrea M, Pliskin N, Barth J, et al. Official position of the military TBI task force on the role of neuropsychology and rehabilitation psychology in the evaluation, management, and research of military veterans with traumatic brain injury. Clin Neuropsychol 2008;22(1):10–26.
88. Department of Veterans Affairs, Department of Defense. VA/DoD clinical practice guidelines for management of concussion/mild traumatic brain injury (mTBI). Available at: http://www.healthquality.va.gov/mtbi/concussion_mtbi_full_1_0.pdf. Accessed August 14, 2013.
89. Jorge RE, Acion L, White W, et al. White matter abnormalities in veterans with mild traumatic brain injury. Am J Psychiatry 2012;169:1284–91.
90. Silver JM. Diffusion tensor imaging and mild traumatic brain injury in soldiers: abnormal findings, uncertain implications. Am J Psychiatry 2012;169(12):1230–2.
91. Ruff RL, Ruff SS, Wang XF. Improving sleep: initial headache treatment in OIF/OEF veterans with blast-induced mild traumatic brain injury. J Rehabil Res Dev 2009;46(9):1071–84.
92. Chard KM, Schumm JA, McIlvain SM, et al. Exploring the efficacy of a residential treatment program incorporating cognitive processing therapy-cognitive for veterans with PTSD and traumatic brain injury. J Trauma Stress 2011;24(3):347–51.
93. Walter KH, Kiefer SL, Chard KM. Relationship between posttraumatic stress disorder and postconcussive symptom improvement after completion of a posttraumatic stress disorder/traumatic brain injury residential treatment program. Rehabil Psychol 2012;57(1):13–7.
94. Wolf GK, Strom TQ, Kehle SM, et al. A preliminary examination of prolonged exposure therapy with Iraq and Afghanistan veterans with a diagnosis of posttraumatic stress disorder and mild to moderate traumatic brain injury. J Head Trauma Rehabil 2012;27(1):26–32.
95. Bryant RA, Moulds M, Guthrie R, et al. Treating acute stress disorder following mild traumatic brain injury. Am J Psychiatry 2003;160(3):585–7.
96. Department of Veterans Affairs, Department of Defense. VA/DoD clinical practice guidelines for management of post-traumatic stress. Available at: http://www.healthquality.va.gov/ptsd/cpg_PTSD-FULL-201011612.pdf. Accessed August 14, 2013.
97. Capehart B, Bass D. Review: managing posttraumatic stress disorder in combat veterans with comorbid traumatic brain injury. J Rehabil Res Dev 2012;49(5):789–812.
98. Raskind MA, Peskind ER, Kanter ED, et al. Reduction of nightmares and other PTSD symptoms in combat veterans by prazosin: a placebo-controlled study. Am J Psychiatry 2003;160(2):371–3.
99. Raskind MA, Peskind ER, Hoff DJ, et al. A parallel group placebo controlled study of prazosin for trauma nightmares and sleep disturbance in combat veterans with post-traumatic stress disorder. Biol Psychiatry 2007;61(8):928–34.
100. Raskind MA, Peterson K, Williams T, et al. A trial of prazosin for combat trauma PTSD with nightmares in active-duty soldiers returned from Iraq and Afghanistan. Am J Psychiatry 2013;170(9):1003–10.

101. Schoefeld FB, Deviva JC, Manber R. Treatment of sleep disturbances in post-traumatic stress disorder: a review. J Rehabil Res Dev 2012;49(5):729–52.
102. Silver JM, McAllister TW, Arciniegas DB. Depression and cognitive complaints following mild traumatic brain injury. Am J Psychiatry 2009;166(6):653–61.
103. Zatzick D, Jurkovich G, Rivara FP, et al. A randomized stepped care intervention trial targeting posttraumatic stress disorder for surgically hospitalized injury survivors. Ann Surg 2013;257(3):390–9.

Sleep and Fatigue Following Traumatic Brain Injury

Jennie L. Ponsford, PhD[a,b,*], Kelly L. Sinclair, DPsych[a,b]

KEYWORDS

- Traumatic brain injury • Fatigue • Sleep disturbance • Depression • Attention
- Treatment

KEY POINTS

- Sleep disturbance and fatigue are common and persistent consequences of traumatic brain injury (TBI), occurring across the spectrum of injury severity.
- Their nature and causes are multifactorial.
- Sleep disturbance may result from damage to sleep-wake regulating centers or from secondary factors, including pain, depression, and anxiety.
- Fatigue may result from impaired attention and speed of information processing, necessitating greater cognitive effort in performing tasks, and secondary factors, including pain, medication, anxiety, and depression, although fatigue may also cause depression and anxiety.
- Assessment of all potential causes is important to determine appropriate treatment.
- Limited research is available demonstrating effective treatment approaches, although trials of both nonpharmacologic and pharmacologic interventions show promising preliminary findings.

Sleep disturbance and fatigue are common consequences of TBI across the spectrum of injury severity. Sleep disturbances have been documented in individuals with mild, moderate, or severe TBI,[1] both in the early stages of recovery[2,3] and in the longer term.[4–9] Fatigue is one of the most common symptoms experienced in the days or weeks after mild TBI and persists in a proportion of cases.[10–12] Fatigue is also reported by up to 70% of individuals with moderate to severe TBI and may continue over many years.[8,13–19] Despite the frequency of subjective complaints of both sleep disturbances and fatigue in individuals with TBI, their nature and causes are not well understood and there are no well-established treatments of these problems. This article discusses the nature, measurement, causes, consequences, and treatments of sleep disturbance and fatigue after TBI.

Disclosure Statement: The authors report no conflicts of interest.
[a] School of Psychological Sciences, Monash University, Melbourne, Australia; [b] Monash-Epworth Rehabilitation Research Centre, Epworth Hospital, Melbourne, Australia
* Corresponding author. School of Psychological Sciences, Building 17, Monash University, Clayton Campus, Victoria 3800, Australia.
E-mail address: jennie.ponsford@monash.edu

Psychiatr Clin N Am 37 (2014) 77–89
http://dx.doi.org/10.1016/j.psc.2013.10.001
0193-953X/14/$ – see front matter © 2014 Elsevier Inc. All rights reserved.

Abbreviations	
TBI	Traumatic Brain Injury
PTA	Post-traumatic Amnesia
EDS	Excessive Daytime Sleepiness
REM	Rapid Eye Movement
MWT	Maintenance of Wakefulness Test
PSQI	Pittsburgh Sleep Quality Index
ESS	Epworth Sleepiness Scale
TMS	Transcranial Magnetic Stimulation
CNS	Central Nervous System
PNS	Peripheral Nervous System
VAS-F	Visual Analogue Scale for Fatigue
FSS	Fatigue Severity Scale
BNI Fatigue Scale	Barrow Neurological Institute Fatigue Scale
GFI	Global Fatigue Index
MAF	Multidimensional Assessment of Fatigue
COF	Causes of Fatigue
COF-ME	Causes of Fatigue-Mental Effort
COF-PE	Causes of Fatigue-Physical Effort
GHD	Growth Hormone deficiency

SLEEP DISTURBANCES AFTER TBI—THEIR NATURE AND ASSESSMENT

Sleep disturbances associated with TBI are broad and may include formally diagnosed sleep disorders (eg, insomnia, hypersomnia, obstructive sleep apnea, periodic limb movements, and narcolepsy) as well as specific complaints (such as snoring, nightmares, poor sleep efficiency, delayed sleep onset, early awakenings, and excessive daytime sleepiness [EDS]) and poorer sleep quality.[1] Makley and colleagues[2,20] reported that up to 68% of individuals were observed to show sleep disruption during acute recovery and early rehabilitation. This disruption was associated with being in posttraumatic amnesia (PTA). Sherer and colleagues[21] found that improvement in daytime arousal and nighttime sleep disturbances preceded improvement in confusion and other acute symptoms during recovery from posttraumatic confusion.

Although there is evidence of resolution of sleep-wake disturbance coincident with emergence from PTA,[22] more chronic sleep difficulties are often reported in the months and years that follow injury.[1,5,9] On average, approximately half of those who sustain TBI experience some form of sleep disturbance, a rate that is significantly higher than in the general community.[1] Insomnia, hypersomnia, and obstructive sleep apnea are considered the most commonly diagnosed sleep disorders after TBI.[1] EDS is also a commonly reported sleep complaint. EDS is manifested as tiredness or drowsiness during the daytime after insufficient sleep or sleep disruption. Although a theoretic distinction exists between EDS and fatigue, the symptoms may not be differentiated by individuals experiencing them.

Estimates of the prevalence of sleep disturbances after TBI seem to vary, however, depending on the type of disturbance and its measurement technique, with objective sleep changes not always consistent with self-reported patterns. Polysomnographic studies have identified longer sleep-onset latencies and increased nighttime awakenings. Some of these studies have also revealed increased slow wave or deep sleep and changes in rapid eye movement (REM) sleep.[23–25] Ouellet and Morin[26] found a higher proportion of stage 1 sleep in a small group of individuals with mild to severe TBI in addition to increased sleep fragmentation. Other studies have not identified any differences in sleep architecture or sleep continuity between individuals with TBI and healthy controls.[27,28] The samples in these studies have been small, however.

Several studies have used actigraphy as an objective measure of sleep in adults after TBI, with reports of poor sleep efficiency in patients in PTA assessed in a subacute rehabilitation setting,[20] increased time spent asleep approximately 6 months postinjury,[4] and identification of circadian rhythm disturbance in individuals with mild TBI.[29] The use of actigraphy to supplement sleep diary reports is recommended, although weaker agreement/consistency between these methods was found in patients with TBI relative to noninjured controls, and further work may be required to understand the accuracy of actigraphy for assessment of sleep disturbance after TBI.[30] Beaulieu-Bonneau and Morin[27] used the Maintenance of Wakefulness Test (MWT) to objectively assess the capacity of individuals with moderate to severe TBI to remain awake during the day. They found no significant differences relative to healthy controls and no association between objectively measured sleepiness on the MWT and either subjective daytime sleepiness assessed using the Epworth Sleepiness Scale (ESS) or fatigue measured on the Multidimensional Fatigue Inventory.

Various self-report measures are available to document sleep difficulties. A systematic review of subjective sleep questionnaires by Mollayeva and colleagues[31] reported that, although no measure met criteria within the well-established to promising ranges, two measures have been more commonly used with reported validity in individuals with TBI. The Pittsburgh Sleep Quality Index (PSQI) is a measure of self-reported sleep quality shown sensitive to sleep disturbance in the TBI population.[1,32] A cutoff score greater than 8 has demonstrated high sensitivity (93%) and specificity (100%) to insomnia in outpatients with TBI.[33] Poorer sleep quality has been documented using the PSQI in individuals with mild to severe TBI.[8,9,34,35] The ESS[36] is widely used in research and clinical practice to identify people with EDS. The ESS requires individuals to rate their likelihood of dozing or falling asleep in specified sedentary situations. A total score greater than or equal to 10 (range 0–24) is considered an indicator of EDS.[36] Recent studies involving individuals with predominantly moderate to severe TBI studied over several years postinjury have reported higher ESS scores in comparison with healthy controls,[9,27] although this has not been a universal finding and may depend on sample size.[27,37]

Other studies have used clinical interview to diagnose sleep disturbances. Baumann and colleagues[4] found that in a group of 65 patients with TBI assessed 6 months postinjury, 47 (72%) had a sleep-wake disturbance, including subjective EDS (28%), objective EDS (25%), fatigue without EDS (17%), hypersomnia (22%), and insomnia (5%). Using a structured diagnostic interview, Cantor and colleagues[8] reported a frequency of diagnosis of insomnia of 11% and 14% in two different groups with moderate to severe TBI recruited from the community at 1 and 2 years postinjury, respectively.

Subjective changes to self-reported sleep have also been examined using sleep diaries. Earlier bedtimes, longer sleep-onset latency, reduced sleep efficiency, greater total sleep duration and time in bed, and longer and more frequent daytime napping have been documented in individuals with mild to severe TBI studied from 3 months to 11 years postinjury in comparison with healthy controls.[7,9,27]

CAUSES OF SLEEP DISTURBANCE AFTER TBI

It seems likely that the causes of sleep disturbances in individuals with TBI are multifactorial. Most of the brain regions, pathways, and neurotransmitter systems associated with sleep regulation, including the suprachiasmatic nucleus, hypothalamus, midbrain, and ascending reticular activating system, are vulnerable to TBI.[4,38] Sleep timing is controlled by the circadian (approximately 24-hour) pacemaker in the hypothalamic suprachiasmatic nuclei, which regulate circadian rhythms. These include the synthesis of melatonin in the pineal gland, which is involved in the circadian regulation of sleep-wakefulness. Although there has not been evidence of changes in dim light melatonin onset, lower levels of evening melatonin production have been identified in individuals with TBI.[25,39] These levels were in turn significantly associated with REM sleep, although not with sleep efficiency or nighttime awakenings.[25] These findings suggest possible disruption of circadian regulation of melatonin synthesis after TBI. Circadian rhythm sleep disorders and delayed circadian timing have been reported in patients with mild TBI and insomnia.[29] Reduced cortical excitability, measured using transcranial magnetic stimulation and similar to that seen in narcolepsy patients, has been associated with objectively measured EDS in a small sample of individuals 3 months after mild to moderate TBI.[40] The investigators hypothesized that this may reflect a deficiency in the excitatory hypocretin/orexin-neurotransmitter system, thought to underpin EDS and hypersomnia in individuals with TBI.[41]

Secondary factors that have been associated with sleep disturbances include pain, depression, and anxiety.[3,5,8,9,35] Greater sleep disturbance 1 year after injury has also been reported by those with multiple comorbidities.[35] Although studies show that depression exacerbates sleep disturbances after TBI, it does not entirely account for them.[25] Another factor having an impact on sleep is fatigue. Fatigue may result in increased frequency of daytime napping, which in turn may have an impact on nighttime sleep quality.[26]

FATIGUE AFTER TBI—ITS NATURE AND ASSESSMENT

Although virtually all people experience fatigue, its definition and measurement present many challenges due to its subjective and multidimensional nature. Aaronson and colleagues[42] have defined fatigue as "The awareness of a decreased capacity for physical and/or mental activity due to an imbalance in the availability, utilization, and/or restoration of resources needed to perform activity." They distinguish between physiologic and psychological sources of fatigue. Physiologic fatigue arises from depletion of energy, hormones, neurotransmitters, or neural connections, in this context due to brain injury. Fatigue that is a result of injury or dysfunction in the central nervous system is termed, *central fatigue*, whereas that caused by malfunction in the peripheral nervous system is termed, *peripheral fatigue*.[43–45] Physical measures of fatigue, such as grip strength or thumb-pressing tasks are more likely to be sensitive to peripheral nervous system dysfunction rather than central fatigue.[45–47] From a psychological point of view, fatigue is defined as "A state of weariness related to reduced motivation, prolonged mental activity, or boredom that occurs in situations such as chronic stress, anxiety or depression."[48] This aspect of fatigue is important to consider, given that anxiety and depression commonly develop after TBI.[49] DeLuca[50] differentiates primary fatigue, which results directly from a disease condition, from secondary fatigue, which is associated with secondary factors, such as pain, sleep disturbance, or mood changes. The subjective experience of fatigue likely represents a combination of these factors.

Several fatigue scales have been developed. These assess various aspects of fatigue, including its severity, its impact on daily activities, and associated feelings. Although no scales have been developed specifically to assess these aspects of fatigue after TBI, several scales have been shown sensitive to fatigue and its effects in this population. The Visual Analogue Scale for Fatigue (VAS-F)[48] quantifies subjective fatigue levels at a single point in time on an 18-item scale, including fatigue and vigor subscales. It has demonstrated reliability and validity. Although the vigor subscale of the VAFS has differentiated head-injured individuals from healthy controls,[47,48] its usefulness in comparison across individuals is limited, because it measures current fatigue from the frame of reference of a single rater. It is, however, potentially useful for examining levels of fatigue or energy within an individual at different times of day or in response to a particular activity or intervention. The Fatigue Severity Scale (FSS)[51] assesses the behavioral consequences of fatigue and the impact of fatigue on daily functioning, rating 9 items on a 7-point scale. The FSS has acceptable internal consistency, stability over time, and sensitivity to clinical changes; discriminates brain-injured patients from controls; and correlates with other fatigue measures.[15,16,47,51] The Barrow Neurologic Institute Fatigue Scale[52] comprises 10 items, such as "How difficult is it for me to maintain my energy throughout out the day?" and "How difficult is it for me to stay alert during activities?" These items are rated on a 7-point scale, with a final item rating overall fatigue on a 10-point scale. Individuals with mild to severe TBI have reported greater fatigue on this scale than healthy controls.[13] The Global Fatigue Index (GFI)[53] is derived from 15 of 16 items of the Multidimensional Assessment of Fatigue. It has established validity and stability in studies of patients with rheumatoid arthritis and has also proved sensitive to fatigue in individuals with brain injury.[17,54] The Causes of Fatigue Questionnaire was developed by Ziino and Ponsford[15] to rate on a 5-point scale the extent to which physical (eg, exercise) and mental (eg, reading and having a conversation) activities cause fatigue. Ziino and Ponsford reported that activities requiring both mental effort and physical effort more frequently caused fatigue in individuals with TBI.[15,16]

There has been little success in the development and validation of objective measures of fatigue in brain-injured populations. Physical measures, such as a thumb-pressing task, have not discriminated brain-injured individuals from controls.[47] Other studies have attempted to demonstrate greater decline in performance over time, either on vigilance tasks or other cognitively demanding tasks. These studies have shown that although overall level of performance was associated with subjective fatigue, there was not a greater decline in task performance over time in groups of individuals with brain injury relative to healthy controls that was associated with subjective fatigue.[54,55] It remains possible that group studies may mask individual differences. The search for an objective marker of fatigue, however, continues.

Studies suggest that fatigue levels may decline somewhat in the first 6 to 12 months postinjury in individuals with moderate to severe TBI but may remain steady or rise slightly thereafter.[16,56] Even as long as 10 years postinjury, a significant proportion of individuals with mild TBI[57] and moderate to severe injuries[19] may continue to report fatigue. There is considerable individual variability, however, across individuals in terms of patterns of fatigue over time.[16] Recent research has also reported on the changing experience of fatigue across a day.[27] Comparing individuals at least 1 year postmoderate to severe TBI to noninjured controls, daytime (hourly) monitoring of fatigue levels using a visual analog scale indicated a progressive increase in self-reported fatigue in the early hours after awakening, whereas a decrease was observed in healthy controls.[27] The potential impact of caffeine restriction during this day on fatigue ratings, however, needs to be considered.

CAUSES OF FATIGUE AFTER TBI

Primary fatigue may result from diffuse neuronal injury, particularly from damage to brain centers that control arousal, attention, and response speed, including the ascending reticular activating system, limbic system, anterior cingulate, and middle frontal and basal ganglia areas.[44,58] Many individuals with brain injury have reduced speed of information processing and experience difficulties with attention, memory, and executive function, which render the performance of cognitively demanding tasks more effortful. van Zomeren and Brouwer[59] contended that fatigue results from the increased effort required to manage daily activities in the presence of cognitive difficulties, including impaired attention and speed of information processing. Impairment of attention and processing speed has been shown associated with subjective fatigue.[54,60] Expending greater effort in performing cognitively demanding tasks results in greater psychophysiologic costs, as reflected by a rise in blood pressure in individuals with TBI that is not evident in healthy controls, that is in turn associated with increased subjective fatigue.[55] These findings support the hypothesis that individuals with brain injury and associated cognitive impairments expend greater effort in performing cognitively demanding tasks, which in turn contributes to subjective fatigue. Arguably the constant need for greater cognitive effort may be stressful for individuals with brain injury.

Some investigators have suggested that fatigue may be associated with neuroendocrine abnormalities after TBI, in particular, that growth hormone deficiency may be associated with fatigue. Growth hormone deficiency is reported in a higher than average proportion of TBI cases.[61,62] Studies have not, however, revealed any significant relationship between pituitary dysfunction and increased fatigue.[34,61,62]

Baumann and colleagues[4] contend that post-TBI fatigue, as well as EDS and hypersomnia, is caused by lower levels of cerebrospinal fluid hypocretin-1, resulting from loss of hypocretin neurons as a consequence of hypothalamic injury. This was supported by findings from a small pathologic study.[38] A decline in hypocretin levels may be associated with increased daytime sleepiness, which may be experienced as fatigue. Hypocretin levels tend to normalize, however, beyond the acute postinjury stages.[41]

There are several potential secondary causes of fatigue. The presence of sleep disturbances may contribute to fatigue, as evidenced by the significant association between these phenomena reported in numerous studies.[16,17,56] Cantor and colleagues[8] found that insomnia without fatigue was rare, whereas fatigue occurred from 21% to 23% of individuals without insomnia.

Increased fatigue has been associated with greater motor deficits.[61] Fatigue has not been related, however, to presence of orthopedic injuries. There is a modest association between fatigue levels and the taking of analgesic medication.[16] Pain levels are also significantly related to subjective fatigue.[14,16,17,61] Higher than average rates of vitamin D deficiency have also been identified in individuals with chronic post-TBI fatigue, presumably due to reduced participation in outdoor activities.[34]

Several studies have reported that depression and anxiety are common in individuals with brain injury who report subjective fatigue.[8,14,16,17,27,61] This relationship may be bidirectional. Although fatigue may be a symptom of depression, experiencing fatigue over long periods may cause depression and anxiety. The authors' recent findings suggest this is the more common occurrence. Schönberger and colleagues[63] found that the presence of fatigue was significantly associated with levels of depression symptoms 6 months later, whereas earlier depression was not associated with the subsequent reporting of fatigue. Cantor and colleagues[17] found that secondary factors accounted for a higher proportion of variance in fatigue in healthy controls than in individuals with brain injury, suggesting that the injury itself may make a unique contribution to fatigue.

With regard to injury and demographic factors, there are trends suggesting that female gender may be associated with higher rates of subjectively reported fatigue,[16,17,61] but demographic factors, such as age or education, or injury-related factors, including injury severity and overall degree of cognitive impairment, show no clear relationships with self-reported fatigue.[13,15–17]

CONSEQUENCES OF FATIGUE AND SLEEP DISTURBANCES

Fatigue and sleep disturbance after TBI often occur in conjunction with cognitive, physical, and emotional changes. Although individually fatigue and sleep disturbance may interact with one another as well as symptoms, such as daytime sleepiness, anxiety, depression, and pain, they also have broader impacts on functional outcome and quality of life. In the inpatient setting, difficulties remaining alert during rehabilitation activities, completing tasks without becoming tired, and staying awake during the day, have been identified.[13]

In the longer term, persisting fatigue and sleep problems may constrain day-to-day living and continue despite apparent physical recovery. These can affect an injured person's ability to engage in domestic activities or complete a full day at work, so that activity levels and productivity are reduced, increased time is spent resting,[27] and there is little energy for social or leisure activities. As a consequence, a pattern of reduced activity and interaction and greater confinement to the home is frequently apparent, even in those with mild injuries.[12] Students may expend greater effort, lose concentration, and have little energy to dedicate to homework as well as other activities.[64] Such lifestyle changes may lead to the development of depression, which may in turn exacerbate fatigue.

Increased reporting of fatigue over time after injury may reflect increased activity levels. There is no demonstrated association, however, between self-reported fatigue and employment status[15,16] or participation in other major life activities.[17] This finding is most likely confounded by individuals who were most impaired also least likely to be employed or engaged in many activities. Nevertheless, fatigue has been shown to make a unique contribution to self-reported disability after injury, as measured on the Mayo-Portland Adaptability Inventory, after controlling for other factors, including executive dysfunction, depression, and injury severity.[65] It has been associated with reduced satisfaction with life in the initial years after injury[8] and up to 15 years later.[17] Individuals with fatigue and sleep disturbance also report poor quality of life.[4,54]

CURRENT TREATMENT APPROACHES

Despite the enduring nature and consequences of fatigue and sleep complaints after TBI, effective treatments are limited. Findings from previously discussed studies may be applied, however, to inform pharmacologic and nonpharmacologic treatment approaches. The multifactorial nature of contributing factors suggests that, in assessing patients who report fatigue or sleep changes, identification, evaluation, and treatment of comorbidities, such as depression, anxiety, and chronic pain, represent appropriate initial steps. Management of underlying medical illness and appropriate treatment of diagnosed sleep disorders (eg, obstructive sleep apnea) are also important.[66]

Nonpharmacologic treatment approaches may include behavioral interventions, psychoeducation, and strategies for management of daytime symptoms as well as psychological therapies. In order to minimize fatigue, individuals with brain injury may need to learn to monitor and adjust their lifestyles to manage within their cognitive and physical limitations. This may involve reducing work hours and work demands, minimizing distraction and necessity for multitasking, and/or building rest breaks into activities. A graduated approach should be taken to increasing activity levels. Individuals who have the ability to control and monitor their behaviors may be taught strategies to cope with information overload and associated social difficulties.

Education in relation to sleep hygiene may also assist in improving nighttime sleep quality. De La Rue-Evans and colleagues[67] reported on a pilot study evaluating a nurse-led sleep hygiene implementation in an inpatient rehabilitation facility for individuals with TBI. Chart reviews preimplementation (n = 34) and postimplementation (n = 33) conducted to assess the impact of the sleep hygiene implementation on self-reported sleep duration did not reveal a statistically significant improvement. The investigators highlighted the importance, however, of sleep hygiene practice in inpatient rehabilitation settings, given the high frequency of reported sleep disturbances. Ouellet and Morin[68] evaluated therapy provided in a case series of individuals with chronic TBI symptoms, including insomnia, who were living in the community. They combined education in sleep hygiene techniques, stimulus control, sleep restriction, and fatigue management with cognitive therapy, encouraging clients to identify, challenge, and alter dysfunctional beliefs and attitudes. Significant reductions in total wake time, sleep efficiency, and reduced fatigue were obtained for 8 (73%) of 11 participants, with progress maintained at 1-month and 3-month follow-ups. Johansson and colleagues[69] found that an 8-week treatment using mindfulness-based stress reduction resulted in significant improvements in mental fatigue in a group of 11 individuals with TBI and/or stroke.

The authors have recently investigated the usefulness of light therapy as a nonpharmacologic approach in alleviating daytime symptoms of fatigue and sleepiness after TBI. Light therapy has the potential not only to increase alertness, thereby reducing fatigue and daytime sleepiness, but also to improve psychomotor vigilance and reduce depression, factors shown associated with fatigue. Findings form a pilot study that has shown a reduction in subjective fatigue and daytime sleepiness in response to this therapy.[70]

Few studies have formally examined the efficacy of pharmacologic treatments in the management of sleep disturbances and fatigue after TBI. Hypnotic and benzodiazepine-like compounds (zolpidem and zopiclone) are not recommended for long-term use in treating insomnia in individuals with TBI. They can be associated with adverse effects, including impaired cognitive function and reduced daytime alertness, hallucinatory behavior, sleepwalking, and altered sleep architecture.[71]

Modafinil is a wake-promoting drug approved in the United States for treating excessive sleepiness in individuals with narcolepsy, obstructive sleep apnea, and shift work disorder. Trials evaluating its use in the TBI population have had mixed findings. Jha and colleagues[72] found no significant reduction in subjective fatigue measured on the FSS in a study of a general TBI sample who did not necessarily present with fatigue or sleep disturbances. They did show, however, a trend toward a reduction in daytime sleepiness in the fourth week, although not in the tenth week of treatment. Another trial of modafinil in 20 people with fatigue/sleepiness problems, conducted by Kaiser and colleagues,[73] showed a reduction in daytime sleepiness but again no impact on fatigue. Johansson and colleagues,[74] investigated the use of a monoaminergic stabilizer, (-)-OSU6162, which has shown some promise in improvement of mental stamina and fatigue in a small group of individuals with acquired brain injury.

Given the authors' findings suggesting that evening melatonin levels may be reduced in individuals with TBI, melatonin supplementation represents another potential treatment of sleep disturbance after TBI. Melatonin has been shown to reduce latency to sleep and increase sleep efficiency in chronic and age-related insomnia.[75,76] One small randomized controlled trial found no significant impact on self-reported sleep parameters of either melatonin or amitriptyline administered over 1 month to 7 men with TBI greater than 6 months postinjury.[77] Melatonin had a moderate effect on daytime alertness compared with amitriptyline, however. The conclusions were limited by a small sample size. Further evaluation of this and other pharmacologic interventions seems warranted.

SUMMARY

Sleep disturbances and fatigue are common and persistent problems after TBI, occurring across the spectrum of injury severity. Although subjective measures of sleep disturbance and EDS can be used in TBI populations, objective sleep studies are important to verify the presence and/or causes of sleep disturbance documented using subjective reports. Common problems include reduced sleep efficiency, increased sleep-onset latency, and/or increased time spent awake after sleep onset. The possibility of reduced melatonin and circadian rhythm disorders may also need to be considered. Anxiety, depression, and pain as well as daytime napping may contribute to sleep difficulties and need to be considered when formulating treatments. Fatigue may be associated with impaired attention and information processing speed, necessitating greater effort in performing tasks. It may also be associated with sleep disturbances, pain, and the taking of analgesic medication as well as depression and anxiety. There is some evidence that fatigue may contribute to depression.

The research evidence to date provides a foundation for development of treatments of fatigue and sleep disturbance after TBI. It is important to assess and treat underlying sleep disorders, such as sleep apnea as well as anxiety, depression, and pain. Injured persons may be supported in making modifications to their lifestyles and daily activities to enable them to live more effectively within their cognitive and physical limitations. Sleep hygiene techniques may assist in minimizing sleep disturbance. There is some preliminary evidence that modafinil may reduce daytime sleepiness. Among nonpharmacologic interventions, light therapy holds promise as a means of increasing daytime alertness as well as enhancing vigilance and mood. Further controlled trials of all of these and other interventions are needed.

REFERENCES

1. Mathias JL, Alvaro PK. Prevalence of sleep disturbances, disorders, and problems following traumatic brain injury: a meta-analysis. Sleep Med 2012;13: 898–905.
2. Makley MJ, English JB, Drubach DA, et al. Prevalence of sleep disturbance in closed head injury patients in a rehabilitation unit. Neurorehabil Neural Repair 2008;22:341–7.
3. Rao V, Spiro J, Vaishnavi S, et al. Prevalence and types of sleep disturbances acutely after traumatic brain injury. Brain Inj 2008;22:381–6.
4. Baumann CR, Werth E, Stocker R, et al. Sleep-wake disturbances 6 months after traumatic brain injury: a prospective study. Brain 2007;130(Pt 7):1873–83.
5. Ouellet MC, Beaulieu-Bonneau S, Morin CM. Insomnia in patients with traumatic brain injury: frequency, characteristics, and risk factors. J Head Trauma Rehabil 2006;21(3):199–212.
6. Kempf J, Werth E, Kaiser PR, et al. Sleep-wake disturbances 3 years after traumatic brain injury. J Neurol Neurosurg Psychiatry 2010;81(12):1402–5.
7. Parcell D, Ponsford J, Rajaratnam S, et al. Self-reported changes to night-time sleep following traumatic brain injury. Arch Phys Med Rehabil 2006;87(2):278–85.

8. Cantor JB, Bushnik T, Cicerone K, et al. Insomnia, fatigue and sleepiness in the first 2 years after traumatic brain injury: an NIDRR TBI Model System Module Study. J Head Trauma Rehabil 2012;27(6):E1–14.
9. Ponsford JL, Parcell DL, Sinclair K, et al. Changes in sleep patterns following traumatic brain injury: a controlled study. Neurorehabil Neural Repair 2013; 27(7):613–21.
10. Ponsford J, Cameron P, Fitzgerald M, et al. Long term outcomes after uncomplicated mild traumatic brain injury: a comparison with trauma controls. J Neurotrauma 2011;28(6):937–48.
11. Lundin A, de Boussard C, Edman G, et al. Symptoms and disability until 3 months after mild TBI. Brain Inj 2006;20(8):799–806.
12. Stulemeijer M, van der Werf S, Bl-ieijenberg G, et al. Recovery from mild traumatic brain injury: a focus on fatigue. J Neurol 2006;253(8):1041–7.
13. Borgaro SR, Baker J, Wethe JV, et al. Subjective reports of fatigue during early recovery from traumatic brain injury. J Head Trauma Rehabil 2005;20(5):416–25.
14. Bushnik T, Englander J, Wright J. The experience of fatigue in the first 2 years after moderate to severe traumatic brain injury: a preliminary report. J Head Trauma Rehabil 2008;23(1):17–24.
15. Ziino C, Ponsford J. Measurement and prediction of subjective fatigue following traumatic brain injury. J Int Neuropsychol Soc 2005;11:416–25.
16. Ponsford JL, Ziino C, Parcell DL, et al. Fatigue and sleep disturbance following traumatic brain injury – Their nature, causes and potential treatments. J Head Trauma Rehabil 2012;27(3):224–33.
17. Cantor JB, Ashman T, Gordon W, et al. Fatigue after traumatic brain injury and its impact on participation and quality of life. J Head Trauma Rehabil 2008;23(1): 41–51.
18. Olver JH, Ponsford JL, Curran C. Outcome following traumatic brain injury: a comparison between 2 and 5 years after injury. Brain Inj 1996;10:841–8.
19. Ponsford JL, Downing M, Olver J, et al. Longitudinal follow-up of patients with traumatic brain injury: outcome at 2, 5, and 10-years post-injury. J Neurotrauma. [Epub ahead of print]. http://dx.doi.org/10.1089/neu.2013.2997.
20. Makley MJ, Johnson-Greene L, Tarwater PM, et al. Return of memory and sleep efficiency following moderate to severe closed head injury. Neurorehabil Neural Repair 2009;23(4):320–6.
21. Sherer M, Yablon SA, Nakase-Richardson R. Patterns of recovery of posttraumatic confusional state in nuerorehabilitation admissions after traumatic brain injury. Arch Phys Med Rehabil 2009;90:1749–54.
22. Nakase-Richardson R, Sherer M, Barnett SD, et al. Prospective evaluation of the nature, course and impact of acute sleep abnormality after traumatic brain injury. Arch Phys Med Rehabil 2013;94:875–82.
23. Orff HJ, Ayalon L, Drummond SP. Traumatic brain injury and sleep disturbance: a review of current research. J Head Trauma Rehabil 2009;24:155–65.
24. Parcell DL, Ponsford JL, Redman JR, et al. Poor sleep quality and changes in objectively recorded sleep after traumatic brain injury: a preliminary study. Arch Phys Med Rehabil 2008;89:843–50.
25. Shekleton JA, Parcell DL, Redman JR, et al. Sleep disturbance and melatonin levels following traumatic brain injury. Neurology 2010;74(21):1732–8.
26. Ouellet MC, Morin CM. Subjective and objective measures of insomnia in the context of TBI. Sleep Med 2006;7(6):486–97.
27. Beaulieu-Bonneau S, Morin CM. Sleepiness and fatigue following traumatic brain injury. Sleep Med 2012;13:598–605.

28. Williams BR, Lazic SE, Ogilvie RD. Polysomnographic and quantitative EEG analysis of subjects with long-term insomnia complaints associated with mild traumatic brain injury. Clin Neurophysiol 2008;119:429–38.

29. Ayalon L, Borodkin K, Dishon L, et al. Circadian rhythm sleep disorders following mild traumatic brain injury. Neurology 2007;68:1136–40.

30. Sinclair K, Ponsford J, Rajaratnam S. Actigraphic assessment of sleep disturbances following traumatic brain injury. Behav Sleep Med. [Epub ahead of print]. http://dx.doi.org/10.1080/15402002.2012.726203.

31. Mollayeva T, Colantonio A, Kenszerska T. Self-report instruments for assessing sleep dysfunction in an adult traumatic brain injury population: a systematic review. Sleep Med Rev 2013;17(6):411–23.

32. Buysse DJ, Reynolds CF 3rd, Monk TH. The Pittsburgh sleep quality index: a new instrument for psychiatric practice and research. Psychiatry Res 1989; 28(2):193–213.

33. Fichtenberg NL, Putnam SH, Mann NR, et al. Insomnia screening in postacute traumatic brain injury: the utility and validity of the Pittsburgh Sleep Quality Index. Am J Phys Med Rehabil 2001;80(5):339–45.

34. Schnieders J, Willemsen D, de Boer H. Factors contributing to chronic fatigue after traumatic brain injury. J Head Trauma Rehabil 2012;27(6):404–12.

35. Fogelberg DJ, Hoffman JM, Dikmen S, et al. Association of sleep and co-occurring psychological conditions at 1 year after traumatic brain injury. Arch Phys Med Rehabil 2012;93(8):1313–8.

36. Johns MW. A new method for measuring daytime sleepiness: the Epworth sleepiness scale. Sleep 1991;14:540–5.

37. Chaumet G, Quera-Salva MA, Macleod A, et al. Is there a link between alertness and fatigue in patients with traumatic brain injury? Neurology 2008;71: 1609–13.

38. Baumann CR, Bassetti CL, Valko PO, et al. Loss of Hypocretin (Orexin) neurons with traumatic brain injury. Ann Neurol 2009;66(4):555–9.

39. Steele DL, Rajaratnam SM, Redman JR, et al. The effect of traumatic brain injury on the timing of sleep. Chronobiol Int 2005;22:89–105.

40. Nardone R, Bergmann J, Kunz A, et al. Cortical excitability changes in patients with sleep-wake disturbances after traumatic brain injury. J Neurotrauma 2011; 28(7):1165–71.

41. Baumann CR, Stocker R, Imhof HG, et al. Hypocretin-1 (orexin A) deficiency in acute traumatic brain injury. Neurology 2005;65:147–9.

42. Aaronson LS, Teel CS, Cassmeyer V, et al. Defining and measuring fatigue. Image J Nurs Sch 1999;31:45–50.

43. Chaudhuri A, Behan PO. Fatigue and basal ganglia. J Neurol Sci 2000;179(1–2): 34–42.

44. Chaudhuri A, Behan PO. Fatigue in neurological disorders. Lancet 2004; 363(9413):978–88.

45. Leavitt VM, DeLuca J. Central fatigue: issues related to cognition, mood and behavior, and psychiatric diagnoses. PM R 2010;2(5):332–7.

46. Walker GC, Cardenas DD, Guthrie MR, et al. Fatigue and depression in brain-injured patients correlated with quadriceps strength and endurance. Arch Phys Med Rehabil 1991;72(7):469–72.

47. LaChapelle DL, Finlayson MA. An evaluation of subjective and objective measures of fatigue in patients with brain injury and healthy controls. Brain Inj 1998;12:649–59.

48. Lee KA, Hicks G, Nino-Murcia G. Validity and reliability of a scale to assess fatigue. Psychiatry Res 1991;36:291–8.

49. Gould KR, Ponsford JL, Johnston L, et al. The nature, frequency and course of psychiatric disorders in the first year after traumatic brain injury, a prospective study. Psychol Med 2011;41(10):2099–109.

50. DeLuca J. Fatigue: its definition, its study, and its future. In: DeLuca J, editor. Fatigue as a window to the brain. Cambridge (MA): The MIT Press; 2005. p. 319–25.

51. Krupp LB, La Rocca NG, Muir-Nash J, et al. The fatigue severity scale: application to patients with multiple sclerosis and systemic lupus erythematosus. Arch Neurol 1989;46:1121–3.

52. Borgaro SR, Kwasnica C, Caples H, et al. Fatigue after brain injury: initial reliability study of the BNI Fatigue Scale. Brain Inj 2004;18:685–90.

53. Borman J, Shively M, Smith TL, et al. Measurement of fatigue in HIV positive adults: reliability and validity of the global fatigue index. J Assoc Nurses AIDS Care 2001;12:75–83.

54. Ashman TA, Cantor JB, Gordon WA, et al. Objective measurement of fatigue following traumatic brain injury. J Head Trauma Rehabil 2008;23(1):33–40.

55. Ziino C, Ponsford J. Vigilance and fatigue following traumatic brain injury. J Int Neuropsychol Soc 2006;12:100–10.

56. Bushnik T, Englander J, Wright J. Patterns of fatigue and its correlates over the first 2 years after traumatic brain injury. J Head Trauma Rehabil 2008;23(1):25–32.

57. Zumstein MA, Moser M, Mottini M, et al. Long-term outcome in patients with mild traumatic brain injury: a prospective observational study. J Trauma 2011;71(1):120–7.

58. Kohl AD, Wylie GR, CGenova HM, et al. The neural correlates of cognitive fatigue intruamtic brain injury using functional MRI. Brain Inj 2009;23(5):420–32.

59. van Zomeren AH, Brouwer WH. Clinical neuropsychology of attention. New York: Oxford University Press; 1994.

60. Ziino C, Ponsford J. Selective attention deficits and subjective fatigue following traumatic brain injury. Neuropsychology 2006;20(3):383–90.

61. Englander J, Bushnik T, Oggins J, et al. Fatigue after traumatic brain injury: association with neuroendocrine, sleep, depression and other factors. Brain Inj 2010;24(12):1379–88.

62. Bushnik T, Englander J, Katznelson L. Fatigue after TBI: association with neuroendocrine abnormalities. Brain Inj 2007;21(6):559–66.

63. Schönberger M, Herrberg M, Ponsford J. Fatigue as a cause, not a consequence of depression and daytime sleepiness: a cross-lagged analysis. J Head Trauma Rehabil. [Epub ahead of print]. http://dx.doi.org/10.1097/HTR.0b013e31829ddd08.

64. Willmott C, Ponsford J, Downing M, et al. Frequency and quality of return to study following traumatic brain injury. J Head Trauma Rehabil, in press.

65. Juengst S, Skidmore E, Arenth PM, et al. Unique contribution of fatigue to disability in community-dwelling adults with traumatic brain injury. Arch Phys Med Rehabil 2013;94(1):74–9.

66. Castriotta RJ, Wilde MC, Lai JM, et al. Prevalence and consequences of sleep disorders in traumatic brain injury. J Clin Sleep Med 2007;3(4):349–56.

67. De La Rue-Evans L, Nesbitt K, Oka RK. Sleep hygiene program implementation in patients with traumatic brain injury. Rehabil Nurs 2013;38(1):2–10.

68. Ouellet MC, Morin CM. Efficacy of cognitive-behavioural therapy for insomnia associated with traumatic brain injury: a single case experimental design. Arch Phys Med Rehabil 2007;88(12):1581–92.

69. Johansson B, Bjuhr H, Ronnback L. Mindfulness-based stress reduction (MBSR) improves long-term mental fatigue after stroke or traumatic brain injury. Brain Inj 2012;26(13–14):1621–8.

70. Sinclair K, Ponsford J, Taffe J, et al. Randomised controlled trial of blue light therapy for fatigue following traumatic brain injury. Neurorehabil Neural Repair. [Epub ahead of print]. http://dx.doi.org/10.1177/1545968313508472.

71. Flanagan S, Greenwald B, Wieber S. Pharamcological treatment of insomnia for individuals with brain injury. J Head Trauma Rehabil 2007;22(1):67–70.

72. Jha A, Weintraub A, Allshouse A, et al. A randomized trial of modafinil for the treatment of fatigue and excessive daytime sleepiness in individuals with chronic traumatic brain injury. J Head Trauma Rehabil 2008;23(1):52–63.

73. Kaiser PR, Valko PO, Werth E, et al. Modafinil ameliorates excessive daytime sleepiness after traumatic brain injury. Neurology 2010;75(20):1780–5.

74. Johansson B, Carlsson A, Carlsson ML, et al. Placebo-controlled cross-over study of the monoaminergic stabiliser (-)-OSU6162 in mental fatigue following stroke or traumatic brain injury. Acta Neuropsychiat 2012;24(5):266–74.

75. Garfinkel D, Laudon M, Nof D, et al. Improvement of sleep quality in elderly people by controlled-release melatonin. Lancet 1995;346(8974):541–4.

76. Zhdanova IV, Wurtman RJ, Regan MM, et al. Melatonin treatment for age-related insomnia. J Clin Endocrinol Metab 2001;86(10):4727–30.

77. Kemp S, Biswas R, Neumann V, et al. The value of melatonin for sleep disorders occuring post-head injury: a pilot RCT. Brain Inj 2004;18(9):911–9.

Neuropsychiatry of Persistent Symptoms After Concussion

Jonathan M. Silver, MD

KEYWORDS

- Concussion • Brain injury • Neuropsychiatry • Chronic symptoms

KEY POINTS

- Symptoms that persist long after a concussion may be the result of multiple factors apart from the actual traumatic brain injury, including neurologic, psychiatric, physical, and psychological factors.
- Evaluation includes careful review of history, medical records, imaging, and neuropsychological tests.
- The presence of psychiatric disorders is often more correlated with continued symptoms than the actual brain injury.
- Certain behavioral dynamics can be activated by a neurologic event, but then take on a life of their own, even when detached from the neurologic cause. Adverse interactions with the insurance and legal system may exacerbate symptoms.
- Psychopharmacologic and other interventions, including exercise, often are beneficial in the treatment of neuropsychiatric symptoms.

INTRODUCTION

Acute postconcussion symptoms are fairly consistent in their presentation, and by definition are time limited. At the initial presentation, the individual complains of feeling fuzzy or slowed down; physical problems including insomnia, fatigue, headache, dizziness and visual problems; and emotional/behavioral problems, including feeling depressed/tearful, anxious, and irritable. Recent consensus statements comprehensively address the initial evaluation of concussion and return to play recommendations.[1,2]

Although most individuals who have been diagnosed with concussion return to baseline functioning within several months, there is a subset of individuals who

Parts of this article have been adapted from Silver JM, Kay T. Persistent symptoms after a concussion. In: Arciniegas DB, Zasler ND, Vanderploeg RD, et al, editors. Management of adults with traumatic brain injury. Washington, DC: American Psychiatric Publishing; 2013. p. 475–500.
Disclosure: Dr J.M. Silver is associate editor for *Journal Watch Psychiatry* and *Up to Date*.
New York University School of Medicine, 40 East 83rd Street, Suite 1E, New York, NY 10028, USA
E-mail address: jonsilver@gmail.com

experience persistent symptoms that affect quality of life. These symptoms may remain in less than 10% of individuals with sports concussions, and are significantly influenced by noninjury-related factors.[3,4] Factors implicated in prolonged symptoms include the pathophysiology of the injury, preinjury factors (such as pre-existing psychiatric and substance use problems, previous traumatic brain injuries (TBIs), intelligence, gender, age, personality style), and postinjury factors (social support, availability of adequate treatment, litigation/compensation).[5,6]

When symptoms spread into multiple domains, persist for more than a few months, and then begin to coalesce and globally impair functioning, it is no longer accurate to use the label postconcussion syndrome. The terms postconcussion syndrome and persistent (or chronic) postconcussion syndrome (or symptoms) are neither valid nor helpful, because symptoms do not represent a single pathophysiologic process.[6] More accurately, these are persistent symptoms that occur after a concussion. TBI is an event, not an explanatory diagnosis. Because multiple factors play a role in the persistence of symptoms that may not reflect a continuation of those first evident after the concussion, it is more accurate to characterize them as persistent symptoms after a concussion, rather than postconcussion syndrome or symptoms.

This article discusses factors that influence the persistence of symptoms after a concussion, and important aspects of evaluation and treatment.

DID A MILD TBI OCCUR?

In assessing late postconcussional symptoms, one must pay close attention to the original event, via both self-report and medical records; neither in isolation is sufficient. However, months or years after the accident, even the diagnosis of TBI may be problematic, even when obtaining history of a mild TBI by screening questions.[7]

Is there evidence, either from loss of consciousness, amnesia, or alteration of consciousness, that disruption of brain functioning occurred? The evolution of symptoms should follow the natural course of recovery after a neurologic injury, and the severity of the symptoms should match the severity of the injury. Symptoms that appear late, or get worse over time, are more likely to contain a non-neurological component, although this does not mean that they are unrelated to the original injury.

Self-report

The patient should be asked to give an unstructured narrative of the event, starting with events leading up to the injury. This may be a more accurate reflection of symptoms than administering a standardized questionnaire.[8] A person will not know if he or she lost consciousness, unless there is a witness, and will most often confuse loss of consciousness with post-traumatic amnesia. This exploration should continue to the point where it is clear that continuous memory has been restored—the cessation of post-traumatic amnesia—taking into account medical interventions (especially sedation and/or analgesic medication). There must be at least an alteration in awareness or a period of confusion to fulfill the minimal criteria for a mild TBI. In addition, the patient's recall of actual events may be inaccurate or even change after multiple iterations, including depositions or seeing pictures.

Medical Records

In many cases, there will be no medical records of the event. Emergency services were not called, or the patient refused treatment. This does not mean that a brain injury did not occur. The medical facts from the acute time period (eg, time for Glasgow Coma Scale (GCS) to return to normal), in combination with the results of brain imaging, may be extremely helpful in estimating the neurologic severity of the event, and therefore the neurologic basis of postconcussional symptoms.

Summary reports of records (such as independent evaluations) may contain inaccuracies, and even the original records may be wrong by either inclusion or error. Emergency room records have been demonstrated to fail to document a large number of brain injuries due to a nonfocused assessment of initial symptoms (patient being dazed or confused) or testing of memory.[9] Records that have the patient being "alert and oriented x3" are not inconsistent with a mild TBI.

Brain Imaging

In most cases of concussion, standard brain imaging modalities (CT, MRI) will be interpreted as normal. Thus, there is a search for more sensitive modalities of brain imaging (3 T MRI, positron emisssion tomography [PET], DTI [Diffusion Tensor Imaging], MRS [Magnetic Resonance Spectroscopy], fMRI [functional MRI]).[10] It is premature to rely on these as "proof" of brain injury, since several questions need to be answered prior to accepting these as routine tests for concussion:

1. What is the frequency of the abnormality in the general population in those without a history of concussion/TBI?
2. What is the natural history of the abnormality (how it changes with time in relationship to the injury, and whether any abnormality persists)?[11]
3. Does the abnormality correlate with symptoms?
4. Can the abnormality be differentiated from the common co-occurring neuropsychiatric conditions, such as anxiety, depression, pain, and migraine headaches?
5. Is there a standardized and uniformly accepted method of analysis? For example, there are several possible ways to analyze a DTI imaging study: whole brain versus

region of interest; statistical group analysis, individual scans or types of lesions,[12,13] and visual versus computer (volumetric analysis).[14]

Before obtaining a study such as DTI, MRS, or PET, one also needs to consider the implications for an abnormal imaging study. At this time, there is no treatment based on an abnormal image. In an analogous situation, studies have demonstrated that for patients with low back pain, there is no relationship between findings on MRI and recovery.[15] An MRI obtained 1 year after surgery or conservative treatment for sciatica and lumbar disc herniation in 283 patients did not distinguish between favorable and unfavorable outcome.[16] Would an abnormal brain imaging study make the person feel more or less optimistic about recovery? Does this depend on the chronicity of the symptoms? For example, would a patient react differently if an abnormal study was obtained 3 months versus 3 years after continuing symptoms?

Neuropsychological Testing

Neuropsychological evaluation may be useful in shedding light on the role of a mild brain injury on functioning. Test performance is human behavior, and is multiply determined, by the patient (including levels of fatigue) and the test administrator (duration, testing environment, and quality of interaction). No neuropsychological test results are interpretable without the validation of tests of effort. There is substantial evidence that performance on tests of effort contributes significantly to the outcome of cognitive testing.[17] Even when tests of effort are passed, factors such as depression, anxiety, fatigue, and persistence may affect test performance. Other factors that may relate to test performance will be discussed.

WHAT IS CAUSING THE SYMPTOMS?

For those patients with persistent symptoms, specific factors need to be addressed, including psychiatric factors, physical factors, psychological factors, legal factors, insurance factors and effort.

Psychiatric Factors

The presence and severity of symptoms after mild TBI are influenced by co-occurring psychiatric disorders, such as depression, anxiety, and PTSD,[18–23] and may be a significant predictor of symptoms. The presence of psychiatric disorders is a major factor in impairing ability to function and symptom exacerbation.[18,19,22] However, during the acute stage, patients with trauma and no TBI may have similar complaints.[24] While the presence of TBI increases the likelihood of post-traumatic stress disorder (PTSD), panic disorder, agoraphobia, and social phobia at 12 months, psychiatric disorder, not TBI, increases the likelihood of self-reported functional impairment.[25]

Depression may impair neuropsychological test performance in some TBI patients. Depression accounted for a significant proportion of both subjective complaints and poor neuropsychological test performance, although even after adjustment for depression, several cognitive problems remain significant.[20] When this group examined the influence of depression on postconcussion symptoms in 200 patients with mild-to-moderate TBI, the depressed group (96 individuals with major depression or depression-like episodes) had worse self-reported symptoms than the nondepressed group in each symptom cluster (mood/cognition, general somatic, and visual somatic).[26]

Some studies have demonstrated that PTSD is more strongly correlated with post-concussive symptoms than is the occurrence of TBI. In a study evaluating soldiers 3 to

4 months after return from deployment regarding occurrence of TBI, data were gathered on physical symptoms, depression, and PTSD. Soldiers reporting a concussion were more likely to have PTSD than were those with no injuries. Loss of consciousness or an altered mental state was associated with an increased risk for PTSD. Although soldiers with mild TBI had poorer general health, the effect (except for headache) was nonsignificant when controlled for PTSD and depression.[21] In a group of veterans, PTSD mediated the relationship between mild TBI and health and psychosocial outcomes.[23] Symptoms of PTSD overlap with symptoms following concussion, and PTSD may occur in situations were a mild brain injury also occurs. It is important, but difficult, for clinicians to sort when symptoms are due to PTSD, and not the lingering effects of brain injury.[27]

Physical Factors

Persons who sustain concussions often suffer other physical injuries (as well as those in accidents who do not have a TBI). These injuries can indirectly lead to brain dysfunction, and can mimic the cognitive deficits of TBI. Somatic symptoms, such as pain, insomnia, and dizziness, produce their own constellation of cognitive, behavioral, and emotional problems. Inner ear damage can result in vestibular damage, and vestibular–visual mismatch, resulting in both imbalance and distress, and interfere with focus, concentration, communication, and memory.[28] Visual problems, including difficulties with accommodation, are common.[29–31] Headaches and nonhead injury-related pain (especially from neck and back injuries sustained concomitantly with a concussion) can interfere acutely with cognitive focus and impairment of attention, processing speed, memory, and executive functions, as well as changes in mood, somatic preoccupation, and sleep disturbances.[32] Both pain and emotional distress commonly lead to sleep deprivation, which reduces cognitive functioning. When sleep disturbance combines with pain and secondary depression, it is virtually impossible to distinguish the effects (until treated) from TBI. Although less common than after more severe TBI, concussions can cause seizure disorders or hypothalamic damage, resulting in hormonal dysregulation.

Psychological Factors

From the time of the injury, expectation of outcome influences prognosis after concussion.[33,34] Thus, whether at the scene of the accident, on a sports sideline, or in the emergency room, psychological factors can play a major role in helping or impeding recovery.

Pre-existing personality style may be a key as to how physical or cognitive changes may trigger emotional dysfunction. In addition to preinjury depressed mood, resilience is a contributor to prolonged symptoms.[35] For example, persons who are chronic overachievers (not high achievers) may deteriorate precipitously if they lose their edge after a concussion (such persons often have strong obsessive–compulsive, perfectionistic traits). Persons with overly strong dependency needs may become passive and withdrawn after an injury that includes a concussion. Trauma in adult life has great potential to reactivate trauma from the past. In persons with a history of sexual or physical abuse, emotional destabilization after relatively mild adult trauma is not uncommon, and can masquerade as brain damage.

Legal Factors, Insurance Factors, and Effort

The adversarial legal and insurance process may worsen the patient's psychological status, and then can inflate the symptoms and entrench the subjective disability. Much has been written about the possible effects of litigation on prolonging disability and symptoms after a concussion.[6] Increased reporting of symptoms, as well as poor results on neuropsychological testing, have been suggested to be the result of litigation and compensation.[36–38] In contrast, several prospective studies have shown that litigation had no effects on the occurrence of depression or PTSD after TBI.[19,39,40] Monetary factors influence behavior, and cheating is common in a normal population.[41] One would expect that the possibility of monetary rewards could influence symptoms after TBI, just as it could influence the opinions rendered in independent evaluations.

However, suboptimal effort and symptom magnification may not be conscious processes.[42] When symptomatic individuals with mild TBI were given cognitively challenging tasks, there was an increase in postconcussive symptoms and autonomic changes associated with decreased speed of processing and subtle memory deficits.[43] Stereotype threat, the observation that a society's view of a subgroup affects its performance, has been demonstrated in many populations (eg, race, gender, age).[44] The anxiety produced by stereotype threat may increase symptoms, and has been demonstrated in nonclinical brain injury groups.[45] Paradoxically, the increased awareness of concussion suffered during sports and in combat may inadvertently increase stereotype threat and could affect performance or the assessment of symptoms in individuals who have sustained a TBI. In this situation, the individual with a TBI will assume the bias that he or she will have difficulties with a cognitive task or will experience certain symptoms associated with the injury, and thus perform poorly on the task or associate symptoms with the TBI.

Studies in behavioral economics reveal that there are costs of anger, loss aversion (where one needs to gain twice as much to offset a loss), and normal cheating that may exacerbate symptoms.[42,46–48] Any evaluation within the insurance and litigation system may engender anger and resentment. In many cases of trauma, the injuries that the individual suffers are never acknowledged by the offender. Interestingly, an apology modulates the need for revenge.[48]

TREATMENT

Treatment begins at the time of the concussion. Education regarding the expected trajectory of symptoms is therapeutic.[49] This initially optimizes the issue of expectation of outcome. One common problem has been the overenthusiastic prescription of rest after concussion. Several days of rest can be beneficial during the period in which there is cerebral metabolic disruption.[50] Evidence suggests that more than this is not beneficial.[51] In fact, the practice of coccooning, where the injured person is told to completely rest for weeks, can be counterproductive, not only deconditioning the person, but giving him or her a heightened sense of vulnerability. The therapeutic use of exercise will be discussed.

Unfortunately, even the confirmation of a concussion will not decide whether the symptoms are solely from the brain injury. The presence of abnormal imaging may lend weight to the suspicion of a concussion, but can, at most, be used for confirmation of the clinical history, and does not influence treatment decisions. Neuropsychological testing will reveal what domains are problematic, and can be consistent with a concussion (especially speed of processing issues), but is not diagnostic. Thus, one is left with a constellation of symptoms that the clinician attempts to tease apart as to etiology and treatment.

Treatment of the patient who continues to be symptomatic months after sustaining a concussion requires a thorough evaluation of possible contributing factors and a comprehensive treatment plan that targets these issues. One clinical key that can be invaluable in deciphering multiple factors can be the response to exercise. An important question is whether the classic concussion symptoms (eg, fogginess, mental heaviness) are exacerbated with even mild aerobic exercise. Willer and Leddy, at at the Sports Concussion Center at the University of Buffalo, have formalized this assessment using a 10-minute treadmill test (same as the Borg protocol for heart disease).[52–54] While pulse rate and blood pressure are monitored, patients are asked about any symptoms experienced. This group has found that 1 group experiences concussion symptoms (eg, head feels heavy, foggy) at a relatively low heart rate. Another group does not have symptom exacerbation, despite obtaining a maximal heart rate. The first group therapeutically responds to a gradual weekly increase in aerobic exercise, starting at a level below the threshold for symptom exacerbation. The second group has been found to have other causes for symptoms, most often musculoskeletal, but also visual or vestibular, and requires specific rehabilitation for these problems.

One important caveat is that this is the experience of 1 research group in sports concussions; these findings need to be duplicated in other centers with more complicated patients.

The presence of multiple other symptoms affects prognosis, and these symptoms often are overlooked by clinicians unfamiliar with TBI. Headaches may be caused by neck and shoulder musculoskeletal problems, and require physical manipulation, in addition to the use of analgesics. Dizziness and vestibular problems may require vestibular therapy.[28,55] Visual problems may result in headaches, exacerbate vestibular symptoms, and require specific treatment.[31,56] All of these treatments are, at one level, in the service of restoring a positive sense of self for the injured person.

Ameliorating neurologic and physical symptoms cannot be the sole focus of treatment. For TBI patients, depression worsens all symptoms, whether typical depressive symptoms (eg, sleep, mood, or concentration) or somatic ones (eg, vision impairments, nausea, headaches, or dizziness). Because of the common co-occurrence of depression and anxiety and the effects that they have on cognition, disability, and return to work, continued efforts at finding an effective treatment must be pursued.[57] Selective serotonin reuptake inhibitors (SSRIs) are usually the first-line medications for depression, but may require other strategies or augmentation. Medications for cognition, fatigue, irritability, and sleep can be useful. For example, this includes the use of stimulants, cholinesterase inhibitors, amantadine, buspirone, and trazodone. Guidelines for the use of medication are found in **Box 1**.

Box 1
Principles of Psychopharmacology in the Patient with Traumatic Brain Injury

- With respect to dosing, "start low and go slow."

- Employ therapeutic trials of all medications.

- Establish a schedule for systematic reassessment of the clinical condition for which treatment is prescribed.

- Monitor for the development of drug–drug interactions.

- Consider augmentation of partial responses to medications.

- Discontinue or lower the dose of the most recently prescribed medication if there is a worsening of the treated symptom soon after the medication has been initiated (or increased).

Two concepts that are of practical importance for the psychological treatment of persistent symptoms, are (1) dysfunctional feedback loops, and (2) the idea that certain behavioral dynamics can be activated by a neurologic event, but then take on a life of their own even when detached from the neurologic cause. A dysfunctional cognitive feedback loop can develop after concussion. A mild TBI occurs, which disrupts cognitive functioning in the short run. In certain individuals, the cognitive slippage and subsequent change in function may elicit fear and anxiety. Anxiety of sufficient magnitude will interfere with cognition in all individuals, and this interference is enhanced when there is a cognitive weak link after a concussion. The increased anxiety heightens the postconcussive cognitive dysfunction, which increases the anxiety, which further interferes with information processing. When depression, sleep disturbance, and/or pain enter the picture, the dysfunctional feedback loop gathers sufficient strength to take on a life of its own. Even when the neurologic effects of the concussion have receded, the patient may continue to exhibit severe cognitive dysfunction. Historically, this dynamic classically evolves and worsens over time. Understanding this dynamic is critical to understanding how the person's sense of self has deteriorated, and is in fact the key to successful intervention.

Although a single uncomplicated mild TBI can result in brain dysfunction, other factors amplify the symptoms. Guidelines for the issues that should be addressed during treatment are found in **Box 2**. Initially, expectations of recovery impact prognosis, and patients should be told that rapid and significant improvement is expected after a concussion.[58] Paradoxically, the increased awareness of concussion suffered during sports and in combat may inadvertently increase stereotype threat. Because depression and anxiety significantly increase symptoms after TBI, they must be actively treated.[57] Trying too hard is counterproductive. Relaxation techniques, slow breathing, and meditation may alleviate anxiety. Mindfulness-based stress reduction may be helpful.[59] Cognitive behavioral therapy may be particularly efficacious in this regard.[60] Slow breathing, at a rate of 5 breaths per minute, may decrease anxiety, and help to correct the abnormality found in heart rate variability after concussion.[61–63]

The author also believes it is useful to discuss the emotional repercussions of the legal and insurance system. Patients need to be informed about the possible adverse effects of the feelings of anger and revenge. The patient's feelings about the cost of the injury need to be explored, as well what he or she believes will be adequate compensation. These have a significant adverse impact on well being. Being sent for an "IME," (Independent Medical Examination) where one knows his or her veracity will be doubted with the implication that one is exaggerating his or her suffering has adverse consequences. The need for justice (which cannot be adequately met) increases anger and resentment, which leads to further depression and anxiety, which exacerbates symptoms. This is a common and self-fulfilling downward spiral. The

---

Box 2
Issues to be Addressed in the Setting of Persistent Symptoms after Concussion

1. Optimize expectations.
2. Treat depression and anxiety.
3. Minimize stereotype threat.
4. Address feelings of anger and revenge.
5. Address loss aversion.
6. Money affects behavior.

patients who do the best seem to have the ability to let the case take its course and go on with their lives, not let the case be their lives. The longer it lasts, the greater the negative emotional cost, and the need for greater compensation.

Sometimes patients with quite mild neurologic deficits never make good recoveries, and continue to rage at the changes in their lives, while other patients with significant impairments learn to find peace. The individual needs to find a way to accept one's self, however that is defined. The physician's role is to assist however possible, along whatever dimensions, in this process of making peace with a new self.

REFERENCES

1. Giza CC, Kutcher JS, Ashwal S, et al. Summary of evidence-based guideline update: evaluation and management of concussion in sports: report of the Guideline Development Subcommittee of the American Academy of Neurology. Neurology 2013;80:2250–7.
2. McCrory P, Meeuwisse W, Aubry M, et al. Consensus statement on concussion in sport—the 4th International Conference on Concussion in Sport held in Zurich, November 2012. Clin J Sport Med 2013;23:89–117.
3. McCrea M, Guskiewicz K, Randolph C, et al. Incidence, clinical course, and predictors of prolonged recovery time following sport-related concussion in high school and college athletes. J Int Neuropsychol Soc 2013;19:22–33.
4. McCrea M, Iverson GL, McAllister TW, et al. An integrated review of recovery after mild traumatic brain injury (MTBI): implications for clinical management. Clin Neuropsychol 2009;23:1368–90.
5. Carroll LJ, Cassidy JD, Peloso PM, et al. Prognosis for mild traumatic brain injury: results of the WHO Collaborating Centre Task Force on Mild Traumatic Brain Injury. J Rehabil Med 2004;84–105.
6. McAllister TW. Mild brain injury. In: Silver JM, McAllister TW, Yudofsky SC, editors. Textbook of traumatic brain injury. 2nd edition. Washington, DC: American Psychiatric Publishing, Inc; 2011. p. 239–64.
7. Vanderploeg RD, Belanger HG. Screening for a remote history of mild traumatic brain injury: when a good idea is bad. J Head Trauma Rehabil 2013;28:211–8.
8. Sullivan KA, Edmed SL. An examination of the expected symptoms of postconcussion syndrome in a nonclinical sample. J Head Trauma Rehabil 2012;27: 293–301.
9. Powell JM, Ferraro JV, Dikmen SS, et al. Accuracy of mild traumatic brain injury diagnosis. Arch Phys Med Rehabil 2008;89:1550–5.
10. Bigler ED. Structural imaging. In: Silver JM, McAllister TW, Yudofsky SC, editors. Textbook of traumatic brain injury. 2nd edition. Washington, DC: APPI; 2011. p. 73–90.
11. Lipton ML, Kim N, Park YK, et al. Robust detection of traumatic axonal injury in individual mild traumatic brain injury patients: intersubject variation, change over time and bidirectional changes in anisotropy. Brain Imaging Behav 2012; 6:329–42.
12. Jorge RE, Acion L, White T, et al. White matter abnormalities in veterans with mild traumatic brain injury. Am J Psychiatry 2013;169:1284–91.
13. Kim NBC, Kim M, Lipton ML. Whole brain approaches for identification of microstructural abnormalities in individual patients: comparison of techniques applied to mild traumatic brain injury. PLoS One 2013;8:e59382.
14. Zhou Y, Kierans A, Kenul D, et al. Mild traumatic brain injury: longitudinal regional brain volume changes. Radiology 2013;267:880–90.

15. Jarvik JG, Hollingworth W, Martin B, et al. Rapid magnetic resonance imaging vs radiographs for patients with low back pain: a randomized controlled trial. JAMA 2003;289:2810–8.

16. el Barzouhi A, Vleggeert-Lankamp CL, Lycklama a Nijeholt GJ, et al. Magnetic resonance imaging in follow-up assessment of sciatica. N Engl J Med 2013;368: 999–1007.

17. Green P. The pervasive influence of effort on neuropsychological tests. Phys Med Rehabil Clin N Am 2007;18:43–68.

18. Fann JR, Katon WJ, Uomoto JM, et al. Psychiatric disorders and functional disability in outpatients with traumatic brain injuries. Am J Psychiatry 1995; 152:1493–9.

19. Rapoport MJ, McCullagh S, Streiner D, et al. The clinical significance of major depression following mild traumatic brain injury. Psychosomatics 2003;44:31–7.

20. Chamelian L, Feinstein A. The effect of major depression on subjective and objective cognitive deficits in mild to moderate traumatic brain injury. J Neuropsychiatry Clin Neurosci 2006;18:33–8.

21. Hoge CW, McGurk D, Thomas JL, et al. Mild traumatic brain injury in US soldiers returning from Iraq. N Engl J Med 2008;358:453–63.

22. Satz P, Forney DL, Zaucha K, et al. Depression, cognition, and functional correlates of recovery outcome after traumatic brain injury. Brain Inj 1998;12:537–53.

23. Pietrzak RH, Johnson DC, Goldstein MB, et al. Posttraumatic stress disorder mediates the relationship between mild traumatic brain injury and health and psychosocial functioning in veterans of operations Enduring Freedom and Iraqi Freedom. J Nerv Ment Dis 2009;197:748–53.

24. Meares S, Shores EA, Taylor AJ, et al. Mild traumatic brain injury does not predict acute postconcussion syndrome. J Neurol Neurosurg Psychiatr 2008;79: 300–6.

25. Bryant RA, O'Donnell ML, Creamer M, et al. The psychiatric sequelae of traumatic injury. Am J Psychiatry 2010;167:312–20.

26. Herrmann N, Rapoport MJ, Rajaram RD, et al. Factor analysis of the Rivermead Post-Concussion Symptoms Questionnaire in mild-to-moderate traumatic brain injury patients. J Neuropsychiatry Clin Neurosci 2009;21:181–8.

27. Stein MB, McAllister TW. Exploring the convergence of post-traumatic stress disorder and mild traumatic brain injury. Am J Psychiatry 2009;166:768–76.

28. Cosetti MK, Lalwani AK. Dizziness, imbalance, and vestibular dysfunctiion. In: Silver JM, McAllister TW, Yudofsky SC, editors. Textbook of traumatic brain injury. 2nd edition. Washington, DC: APPI; 2011. p. 351–61.

29. Green W, Ciuffreda KJ, Thiagarajan P, et al. Accommodation in mild traumatic brain injury. J Rehabil R D 2010;47:183–99.

30. Ciuffreda KJ, Kapoor N, Rutner D, et al. Occurrence of oculomotor dysfunctions in acquired brain injury: a retrospective analysis. Optometry 2007;78:155–61.

31. Kapoor N, Ciuffreda KJ. Vision problems. In: Silver JM, McAllister TW, Yudofsky SC, editors. Textbook of traumatic brain injury. 2nd edition. Washington, DC: APPI; 2011. p. 363–74.

32. Zasler ND, Martelli MF, Nicholson K. Chronic pain. In: Silver JM, McAllister TW, Yudofsky SC, editors. Textbook of traumatic brain injury. 2nd edition. Washington, DC: APPI; 2011. p. 375–96.

33. Whittaker R, Kemp S, House A. Illness perceptions and outcome in mild head injury: a longitudinal study. J Neurol Neurosurg Psychiatr 2007;78:644–6.

34. Mittenberg W, DiGiulio DV, Perrin S, et al. Symptoms following mild head injury: expectation as aetiology. J Neurol Neurosurg Psychiatr 1992;55:200–4.

35. McCauley SR, Wilde EA, Miller ER, et al. Preinjury resilience and mood as predictors of early outcome following mild traumatic brain injury. J Neurotrauma 2013;30:642–52.
36. Tsanadis J, Montoya E, Hanks RA, et al. Brain injury severity, litigation status, and self-report of postconcussive symptoms. Clin Neuropsychol 2008;22: 1080–92.
37. Binder LM, Rohling ML. Money matters: a meta-analytic review of the effects of financial incentives on recovery after closed-head injury. Am J Psychiatry 1996; 153:7–10.
38. Paniak C, Reynolds S, Toller-Lobe G, et al. A longitudinal study of the relationship between financial compensation and symptoms after treated mild traumatic brain injury. J Clin Exp Neuropsychol 2002;24:187–93.
39. Deb S, Lyons I, Koutzoukis C, et al. Rate of psychiatric illness 1 year after traumatic brain injury. Am J Psychiatry 1999;156:374–8.
40. Koren D, Arnon I, Klein E. Acute stress response and posttraumatic stress disorder in traffic accident victims: a one-year prospective, follow-up study. Am J Psychiatry 1999;156:367–73.
41. Ariely D. Predictably irrational, revised and expanded edition: the hidden forces that shape our decisions. New York: Harper Collins; 2009.
42. Silver JM. Effort, exaggeration and malingering after concussion. J Neurol Neurosurg Psychiatr 2012;83:836–41.
43. Hanna-Pladdy B, Berry ZM, Bennett T, et al. Stress as a diagnostic challenge for postconcussive symptoms: sequelae of mild traumatic brain injury or physiological stress response. Clin Neuropsychol 2001;15:289–304.
44. Steele CM. Whistling Vivaldi: and other clues to how stereotypes affect us. New York: W.W. Norton & Co; 2010.
45. Pavawalla SP, Salazar R, Cimino C, et al. An exploration of diagnosis threat and group identification following concussion injury. J Int Neuropsychol Soc 2013; 19:305–13.
46. de Quervain DJ, Fischbacher U, Treyer V, et al. The neural basis of altruistic punishment. Science 2004;305:1254–8.
47. Kahneman D, Tversky A. Prospect theory: an analysis of decision under risk. Econometrica 1979;47:263–91.
48. Ariely D. The upside of irrationality. The unexpected benefits of defying logic at work and at home. New York: Harper Collins; 2010.
49. Larson EB, Kondiles BR, Starr CR, et al. Postconcussive complaints, cognition, symptom attribution and effort among veterans. J Int Neuropsychol Soc 2013; 19:88–95.
50. Giza CC, Hovda DA. The neurometabolic cascade of concussion. J Athl Train 2001;36:228–35.
51. Silverberg ND, Iverson GL. Is rest after concussion "the best medicine?" Recommendations for activity resumption following concussion in athletes, civilians, and military service members. J Head Trauma Rehabil 2013;28:250–9.
52. Leddy JJ, Kozlowski K, Donnelly JP, et al. A preliminary study of subsymptom threshold exercise training for refractory post-concussion syndrome. Clin J Sport Med 2010;20:21–7.
53. Leddy JJ, Baker JG, Kozlowski K, et al. Reliability of a graded exercise test for assessing recovery from concussion. Clin J Sport Med 2011;21:89–94.
54. Leddy JJ, Cox JL, Baker JG, et al. Exercise treatment for postconcussion syndrome: a pilot study of changes in functional magnetic resonance imaging activation, physiology, and symptoms. J Head Trauma Rehabil 2013;28:241–9.

55. Gurr B, Moffat N. Psychological consequences of vertigo and the effectiveness of vestibular rehabilitation for brain injury patients. Brain Inj 2001;15:387–400.
56. Ciuffreda KJ, Rutner D, Kapoor N, et al. Vision therapy for oculomotor dysfunctions in acquired brain injury: a retrospective analysis. Optometry 2008;79: 18–22.
57. Silver JM, McAllister TW, Arciniegas DB. Depression and cognitive complaints following mild traumatic brain injury. Am J Psychiatry 2009;166:653–61.
58. Wade DT, King NS, Wenden FJ, et al. Routine follow-up after head injury: a second randomised controlled trial. J Neurol Neurosurg Psychiatr 1998;65:177–83.
59. Azulay J, Smart CM, Mott T, et al. A pilot study examining the effect of mindfulness-based stress reduction on symptoms of chronic mild traumatic brain injury/postconcussive syndrome. J Head Trauma Rehabil 2013;28:323–31.
60. Hou R, Moss-Morris R, Peveler R, et al. When a minor head injury results in enduring symptoms: a prospective investigation of risk factors for postconcussional syndrome after mild traumatic brain injury. J Neurol Neurosurg Psychiatr 2011;83(2):217–23.
61. Gall B, Parkhouse W, Goodman D. Heart rate variability of recently concussed athletes at rest and exercise. Med Sci Sports Exerc 2004;36:1269–74.
62. Tharion E, Samuel P, Rajalakshmi R, et al. Influence of deep breathing exercise on spontaneous respiratory rate and heart rate variability: a randomised controlled trial in healthy subjects. Indian J Physiol Pharmacol 2012;56:80–7.
63. Vaschillo E, Lehrer P, Rishe N, et al. Heart rate variability biofeedback as a method for assessing baroreflex function: a preliminary study of resonance in the cardiovascular system. Appl Psychophysiol Biofeedback 2002;27:1–27.

Apathy Following Traumatic Brain Injury

Sergio E. Starkstein, MD, PhD[a],*, Jaime Pahissa, MD[b]

KEYWORDS

- Apathy • Traumatic brain injury • Depression • Cognitive deficits
- Psychotropic medication • Psychotherapy

KEY POINTS

- Apathy is a frequent behavioral complication of traumatic brain injury (TBI) and may be present in at least half of patients at some stage of the post-TBI period.
- One of the most important limitations to diagnose apathy in TBI is the lack of specific scales to rate the severity of this condition in TBI and the lack of validated diagnostic criteria.
- Apathy in TBI is significantly associated with both depression and cognitive impairments but may also present as an independent phenomenon. One of the major complications of apathy in TBI is its negative impact on rehabilitation efforts.
- Anecdotal evidence suggests that psychostimulant medication may be of use in some patients with TBI, and there is an urgent need for proper randomized controlled trials for pharmacotherapy and psychotherapy to be conducted in TBI.

INTRODUCTION

Traumatic brain injury (TBI) may result in significant emotional and behavioral changes, such as depression, impulsivity, anxiety, aggressive behavior, and posttraumatic stress disorder.[1] Apathy has been increasingly recognized as a relevant sequela of TBI, with a negative impact on the patients' quality of life as well as their participation in rehabilitation activities. This article reviews the nosologic and phenomenological aspects of apathy in TBI, diagnostic issues, frequency and prevalence, relevant comorbid conditions, potential mechanisms, and treatment.

APATHY: DEFINITION AND PHENOMENOLOGY

Marin[2] was the first to suggest apathy as an independent neuropsychiatric syndrome describing apathy as a general reduction in motivation. Apathy was operationalized as

Disclosures: The authors have nothing to disclose.
[a] School of Psychiatry and Clinical Neurosciences, University of Western Australia, Fremantle Hospital T-7, Fremantle, Western Australia 6959, Australia; [b] Department of Psychiatry, CEMIC University, Valdenegro 4337, Buenos Aires 1430, Argentina
* Corresponding author.
E-mail address: sergio.starkstein@uwa.edu.au

Psychiatr Clin N Am 37 (2014) 103–112
http://dx.doi.org/10.1016/j.psc.2013.10.002
0193-953X/14/$ – see front matter Crown Copyright © 2014 Published by Elsevier Inc. All rights reserved.

Abbreviations	
TBI	Traumatic Brain Injury
DSM 5	Diagnostic and Statistical Manual-fifth edition
ICD-10	International Classification of Diseases -10th edition
SCIA	Structured Clinical Interview for Apathy
AES	Apathy Evaluation Scale
LARS	Lille Apathy Rating Scale
FrSBe	Frontal System Behaviour Scale
NPI	Neuropsychiatry Inventory
MRI	Magnetic Resonance Imaging
DTI	Diffusion Tensor Imaging

reductions in goal-directed behaviors (eg, lack of effort, initiative, and productivity), reductions in goal-directed cognitions (eg, decreased interests, lack of plans and goals and lack of concern about one's own health or functional status), and reduced emotional concomitants of behaviors (eg, flattened affect, emotional indifference, and restricted responses to important life events).[3] Other definitions of apathy stress the emotional deficits,[4] such as absence of feelings with blunting and flattening of affective response. Levy and Dubois[5] focused on the behavioral deficits and defined apathy as an observable behavioral syndrome characterized by a quantitative reduction of self-generated voluntary and purposeful behaviors. They suggested 3 subtypes of apathy: emotional-affective, cognitive, and auto-activation. These behavioral deficits should occur in the absence of contextual or physical changes and should be reversed by external stimulation.

In conclusion, important questions remain unanswered regarding the nosologic position of apathy in neuropsychiatric conditions. It is unclear whether apathy should be considered a symptom or a syndrome, and it has yet to be included in the major psychiatric nomenclatures. Apathy is sometimes considered a deficit of motivation, a blunted emotional state, or a behavioral deficit excluding psychological components.

DIAGNOSIS OF APATHY

Apathy should be diagnosed only after a thorough psychiatric assessment including the evaluation of the individual's social and physical context. Marin and Wilkosz[6] made the important clarification that individuals greatly differ in terms of their goals, interests, and pattern of emotional display, which are all strongly related to relevant demographic factors, such as level of education, type of upbringing, social class, and age cohort. In the TBI rehabilitation setting, important factors, such as role loss, motor and sensory deficits, and cognitive impairments, can all impact on the patients' motivation to engage in activities.[7]

Apathy is not listed as a specific syndrome or symptom in either the *Diagnostic and Statistical Manual of Mental Disorders* (Fifth Edition) (*DSM-5*)[8] or the *International Classification of Diseases, Tenth Revision*.[9] Nevertheless, relevant phenomenological information has been collected during the past 2 decades; both Starkstein and Leentjens[10] and the European Psychiatric Association[11] proposed specific diagnostic criteria for apathy for use in neuropsychiatry (**Box 1**). The European criteria are similar to Starkstein and Leentjens', with 2 main differences: (1) they require symptoms from at least 2 of the 3 domains and the rather unclear concept that changes in motivation or emotion may be internally or externally generated.

Box 1
Diagnostic criteria for apathy

1. There is a lack of motivation relative to the patients' previous level of functioning or the standards of their age and culture as indicated either by subjective account or observation by others.

2. There is the presence, *for at least 4 weeks during most of the day,* of at least 1 symptom belonging to each of the following 3 domains:

   Diminished goal-directed behavior

   a. Lack of effort or energy to perform everyday activities

   b. Dependency on prompts from others to structure everyday activities

   Diminished goal-directed cognition

   c. Lack of interest in learning new things or in new experiences

   d. Lack of concern about one's personal problems

   Diminished concomitants of goal-directed behavior

   e. Unchanging or flat affect

   f. Lack of emotional responsivity to positive or negative events

3. The symptoms cause clinically significant distress or impairment in social, occupational, or other important areas of functioning.

4. The symptoms are not caused by a diminished level of consciousness or the direct physiologic effects of a substance.

Adapted from Starkstein S, Leentjens AF. The nosologic position of apathy in clinical practice. J Neurol Neurosurg Psychiatr 2008;79:1088–92; with permission.

Mental status examinations should be ideally carried out with semistructured psychiatric interviews specifically validated for the syndrome under study. To the authors' knowledge, the Structured Clinical Interview for Apathy[12] is the only semistructured clinical interview validated for use in neuropsychiatry. This instrument showed strong psychometric attributes for use in dementia[12] but has to be validated in acute neurologic conditions.

There are several severity rating scales that have been validated for use in neuropsychiatric disorders. Marin and coworkers[13] developed the Apathy Evaluation Scale (AES), an 18-item instrument that can be administered as a self-rating scale, a caregiver rating scale, or a clinician administered test. This scale has been used in most studies of apathy in TBI.[14] Glenn and coworkers[15] examined the psychometric attributes of the AES self-rating and informant versions using a clinical diagnosis of apathy as the gold standard. The researchers were unable to find a cutoff score with adequate sensitivity and specificity in this population, and further validation studies are needed.

The Apathy Scale[16] is an abridged version of Marin's scale and can be rated by patients or an informant. The Children's Motivation Scale[2] is also based on Marin's AES and rates the severity of apathy among children and adolescents. Other scales have been designed for use in specific neurologic disorders, such as the Dementia Apathy and Interview Rating[17] to assess apathy among demented individuals; the Apathy Inventory (AI),[18] which was validated for use in Alzheimer and Parkinson disease; and the Lille Apathy Rating Scale (LARS),[19] which was validated for use in Parkinson disease (PD). The AI is based on the format of the Neuropsychiatry Inventory, assessing both the frequency and severity of apathy in patients and caregivers. The LARS assesses reduction in everyday productivity, lack of interest, lack of initiative, extinction of novelty seeking and motivation, blunting of emotional responses, lack of concern, and poor social life. The Frontal System Behavior Scale[20] was designed to assess and quantify the domains of disinhibition, apathy, and executive dysfunction. In a recent study, Niemeier and coworkers[21] examined the psychometric attributes of the scale in an acute TBI sample. Although the scale showed good internal consistency and reliability, a factor analysis was unable to produce the 3 dimensions described earlier. The Neuropsychiatry Inventory (NPI)[22] is a multidimensional instrument that is administered to caregivers who are familiar with the patients and includes a specific subscale to rate apathy. The final score is based on the frequency and severity of apathy symptoms, such as loss of interest; lack of motivation; decreased spontaneity, affection, and enthusiasm; loss of emotions; and loss of interest in starting new activities. Lane-Brown and Tate[23] suggested that the use of informants to rate apathy has the limitation of not considering subjective aspects of this dimension, and they suggested obtaining reports from patients and multiple informants.

Ambulatory actigraphy was proposed to help in diagnosing apathy in a more ecological way.[24] This technique consists in wearing a wrist device that measures locomotor activity during the daytime. Muller and coworkers[24] assessed with ambulatory actigraphy 24 patients with acquired brain damage and 12 healthy controls. Half of the patients met the diagnostic criteria for a personality change caused by a medical condition (apathetic type), and the other 12 had no apathy or only mild apathy. The main finding was that the activity counts were significantly lower and periods with no activity significantly more frequent in the high-apathy group as compared with the no/mild-apathy and the healthy control groups. Moreover, patients with high apathy took more frequent naps and had shorter activity episodes, mostly in the afternoon. Given that all patients participated in a rehabilitation program with a similar schedule, the researchers concluded that differences obtained with ambulatory actigraphy may provide useful and valid observer-independent quantification of locomotor activity as a proxy for apathy.

In conclusion, there are now reliable and valid scales to rate the severity of apathy in neuropsychiatric conditions. Nevertheless, these instruments still have to be validated for use in TBI. Alternatively, a specific scale to measure the dimension of apathy in TBI should be created.

APATHY IN TBI: DIFFERENTIAL DIAGNOSIS

Several terms have been used to refer to a lack of motivation, blunted affect, and flat emotions. *Abulia* was defined as "the loss, lack, or impairment of the power of the will to execute what is in mind."[25] Marin[26] considered abulia as a more severe expression of apathy. Psychic akinesia has been described in patients that are fully conscious and able to perform their basic activities of daily living but only after strong external stimulation.[27] A similar syndrome that can be reversed by external stimulation has been described by Laplane and Dubois[28] and termed the *autoactivation deficit*. These patients show inertia (ie, the tendency to stay immobile for relatively long periods), mental emptiness, repetitive and stereotyped activities, flat affect, and blunted emotional responses. *Athymormia* (from the Greek *thumos* [mood] and *horme* [impulse]) was coined by Habib[29] to refer to a major reduction in spontaneous motion and speech. Finally, *akinetic mutism* is defined as the inability to initiate actions in patients who appear alert.[4] This state is characterized by a lack of voluntary movement, mutism, and vigilant gaze.[4] Marin and Wilkosz[6] proposed the term "disorders of diminished motivation" to include akinetic mutism, abulia, and apathy in a continuum of decreasing severity. Finally, despair and demoralization occur among individuals with no underlying psychiatric disorders when confronted with relevant stressors in their personal and social environment.[26]

FREQUENCY OF APATHY IN TBI

The frequency of apathy in TBI has been reported to range from 20%[30] to 72%.[31] This wide discrepancy may be explained by sampling biases, the use of different instruments to rate the severity of apathy, and the lack of standardized diagnostic criteria. In one of the initial studies, Kant and coworkers[1] assessed a series of 83 patients with TBI who were referred to a neuropsychiatric clinic. They found that 71% had AES scores in the apathy range, most of them with comorbid depression. The referral bias could have accounted for the high frequency of apathy in this sample. Based on prevalence rate studies reported in the literature, van Reekum and coworkers[32] calculated that 61% of the TBI population have apathy. A recent study by Ciurli and coworkers[33] included 120 individuals with severe TBI who were assessed with the NPI. Apathy was reported in 42% of the sample but usually coexisted with other neuropsychiatric disorders.

APATHY, DEPRESSION, AND COGNITIVE IMPAIRMENT

During the past 2 decades, an increasing number of empiric studies among patients with both neurodegenerative (eg, Alzheimer disease, Parkinson disease) and acute neurological conditions (eg, stroke and TBI) reported a major overlap between apathy and depression.[12,16,34,35] One conceptual reason for this overlap is that depression may be diagnosed based on *DSM-IV* criteria in the absence of depressed mood provided the symptoms of loss of interest or anhedonia are present. Starkstein[36] and coworkers[16] reported that apathy can be validly separated from depression in both Alzheimer disease (AD) and PD. A major overlap between apathy and depression has been reported in TBI. Kant and coworkers[1] assessed 83 consecutive patients with TBI who were evaluated at a neuropsychiatric clinic with the AES and the Beck Depression Inventory (BDI). They found that 71% of the patients met the AES cutoff score for apathy, but only 11% had apathy without depression. In a study that included 28 patients with TBI, Andersson and coworkers[37] reported that among nondepressed participants, 28% had apathy, whereas 59% of the patients with mild depression and 80% of patients with severe depression had apathy. Glenn and coworkers[15] assessed 45 patients with TBI with the AES and the BDI and found significant correlations between the apathy and depression scales.

Marin[26] suggested that apathy should not be diagnosed in the context of moderate or severe cognitive deficits. Several studies have demonstrated an increasing frequency of apathy among patients with increasing levels of cognitive decline.[10,38] Nevertheless, cognitive deficits are not sufficient to produce apathy; about half of the patients with moderate or severe dementia were reported not to have apathy.[10,38]

CORRELATES OF APATHY AFTER TBI

Initial studies found no association between the severity of apathy and TBI.[39] On the other hand, a recent study by Ciurli and coworkers[33] reported that patients with TBI with a functional status recovery score indicating severe disability on the Glasgow Outcome Scale had 4 times the risk of developing apathetic behaviors than patients with TBI with less severe scores. Rao and coworkers[40] examined clinical and demographic correlates of apathy among patients with a first-ever TBI. Fifty-seven percent of the sample had mild TBI, whereas the rest had moderate or severe TBI. The main finding was that apathy at baseline was associated with increased sleep disturbance 12 months after the TBI. On the other hand, baseline apathy was not associated with apathy 1 year later. Andersson and Bergedalen[39] found a significant association between more severe apathy and acquisition and recall memory deficits, executive dysfunction, and psychomotor speed.

MECHANISM OF APATHY IN TBI

In a study that included patients with TBI and patients with stroke lesions, Paradiso and coworkers[41] reported that patients with dorsolateral prefrontal lesions had a greater reduction of motivation than patients with medial prefrontal damage. On the other hand, in a series of patients with stroke lesions or TBI, Finset and Andersson[42] reported a significant association between more severe apathy and subcortical damage.

In a recent study, Knutson and coworkers[43] examined the neural correlates of apathy using voxel-based lesion mapping in a study that included 176 brain-injured male Vietnam War veterans and 52 uninjured veteran controls. Apathy was diagnosed with the apathy section of the NPI. The main finding was that damage to specific brain regions, such as the left frontal lobe, the supplementary motor region, the anterior cingulate, and the insula, as well as the white matter in the corona radiata and corpus callosum were significantly associated with more severe apathy. However, there was no significant difference in depression scores between participants with lesions associated with apathy and participants with lesions in other brain areas. Based on these findings, the researchers suggested that apathy may be caused by reduced motivation from lesions to the anterior cingulate region. A greater volume of brain loss among participants with apathy as compared with those without apathy may have at least partially accounted for the findings.

Spalletta and coworkers[44] examined with high-resolution magnetic resonance imaging and diffusion tensor imaging (DTI) a series of 72 healthy adults to assess imaging correlates of incipient apathy symptoms. The main finding was a positive correlation between mean diffusivity values and apathy scale scores in the thalami. This association was significant for female but not for male subjects. The correlation between apathy scores and mean diffusivity values were mostly localized in thalamic sections projecting to prefrontal and premotor areas. The researchers also found a significant negative correlation between low fractional anisotropy and increasing apathy scores in the left middle cerebellar peduncle, internal capsule, anterior thalamic radiations, right supramarginal gyrus, right and left occipital lobe, corpus callosum, and left superior temporal area. These significant findings were limited to the female group.

Although the mechanism of apathy after TBI remains unknown, it is likely that the dysfunction of arousal systems may play an important role. Goldfine and Schiff[45] recently reviewed the role of arousal in motor recovery. They discussed research evidence suggesting an arousal system consisting of glutamatergic and cholinergic neurons in the dorsal tegmentum of the midbrain and pons, which activate cortical regions via the basal forebrain bundle and the intralaminar thalamic nuclei. The main cortical regions involved in arousal regulation are the medial frontal and anterior cingulate as well as the multimodal parietal regions. The researchers suggested that brain injuries to this system may impair goal-directed behavior. Andersson and coworkers[37] examined the association between apathy and psychophysiological reactivity (as measured with heart rate variation and electrodermal activity) in 72 patients with acute brain damage (28 patients had a history of TBI). There was a significant inverse correlation between apathy score and heart rate reactivity while patients were performing tests with stress conditions, suggesting that apathy and emotional flattening are physiologically related.

TREATMENT OF APATHY IN TBI

There are unfortunately no studies of pharmacologic or psychological treatment of apathy using adequate methodological standards. Lane-Brown and Tate[23] examined the results of 28 studies that included individuals older than 16 years with an acquired brain injury treated with pharmacologic or cognitive interventions. Most studies used psychostimulants (mostly methylphenidate[23]), dopamine agonists (eg, amantadine and selegiline),[46,47] and acetylcholinesterase inhibitors.[48] All of them included either single patients or small samples, and proper randomized-controlled trials (RCTs) that are adequately powered are still lacking. Muller and von Cramon[49] used bromocriptine in 15 patients with TBI with behavioral problems, including apathy, but results were heterogeneous. Gualtieri and Evans[50] treated 15 patients with methylphenidate in the context of a small controlled trial and noted significant short-term improvements in apathy. Kant and Smith-Seemiller[7] found significant improvements on the AES scores in 18 patients with TBI treated with methylphenidate (N = 10), dextroamphetamine (N = 8), or amantadine (N = 1). The researchers stated that positive results were still maintained after an average of 12 months of follow-up.

A Cochrane systematic review evaluating pharmacologic and psychological interventions for apathy after TBI[23] was only able to include a single trial meeting the inclusion criteria. That was a study using cranial electrotherapy stimulation to decrease inertia after TBI, which showed negative results.[51]

The assessment of behavioral interventions to treat apathy in TBI is still lacking. Kant and Smith-Seemiller[7] recommended including strategies to help patients initiate activities, such as verbal reminders from caretakers, messaging with audiotapes, or visual cues.

In conclusion, there is a lack of proper RCTs for apathy in TBI. Although small case series and case reports suggest some usefulness for psychostimulants, their efficacy and safety have to be properly demonstrated. Psychotherapies tailored to patients' needs may prove a useful option, especially for patients that may not want to take medication or have side effects; but proper studies have yet to be conducted.

SUMMARY

Apathy is a frequent behavioral complication of TBI and may be present in at least half of the patients at some stage of the post-TBI period. One of the most important limitations to diagnose apathy in TBI is the lack of specific scales to rate the severity of this condition and the lack of validated diagnostic criteria. Apathy in TBI is significantly associated to both depression and cognitive impairments but may also present as an independent phenomenon. One of the major complications of apathy in TBI is its negative impact on rehabilitation efforts. Anecdotal evidence suggests that psychostimulant medication may be of use in some patients with TBI, and there is an urgent need for proper RCTs for pharmacotherapy and psychotherapy to be conducted.

REFERENCES

1. Kant R, Duffy JD, Pivovarnik A. Prevalence of apathy following head injury. Brain Inj 1998;12:87–92.

2. Marin RS. Apathy: a neuropsychiatric syndrome. J Neuropsychiatry Clin Neurosci 1991;3:243–54.
3. Starkstein S, Leentjens AF. The nosological position of apathy in clinical practice. J Neurol Neurosurg Psychiatr 2008;79:1088–92.
4. Sims A. Symptoms in the mind. London: Saunders; 2003.
5. Levy R, Dubois B. Apathy and the functional anatomy of the prefrontal cortex-basal ganglia circuits. Cereb Cortex 2006;16:916–28.
6. Marin RS, Wilkosz PA. Disorders of diminished motivation. J Head Trauma Rehabil 2005;20:377–88.
7. Kant R, Smith-Seemiller L. Assessment and treatment of apathy syndrome following head injury. NeuroRehabilitation 2002;17:325–31.
8. American Pstchiatric Association. Diagnostic and statistical manual of mental disorders. 5th edition. Arlington (VA): American Psychiatric Association; 2013.
9. World health Organization. The ICD-10 classification of mental and behavioural disorders. Geneva (Switzerland): WHO; 1993.
10. Starkstein SE, Leentjens AF. The nosological position of apathy in clinical practice. J Neurol Neurosurg Psychiatr 2008;79:1088–92.
11. Robert P, Onyike CU, Leentjens AF, et al. Proposed diagnostic criteria for apathy in Alzheimer's disease and other neuropsychiatric disorders. Eur Psychiatry 2009;24:98–104.
12. Starkstein SE, Ingram L, Garau ML, et al. On the overlap between apathy and depression in dementia. J Neurol Neurosurg Psychiatr 2005;76:1070–4.
13. Marin RS, Biedrzycki RC, Firinciogullari S. Reliability and validity of the apathy evaluation scale. Psychiatry Res 1991;38:143–62.
14. Arnould A, Rochat L, Azouvi P, et al. A multidimensional approach to apathy after traumatic brain injury. Neuropsychol Rev 2013;23:210–33.
15. Glenn MB, Burke DT, O'Neil-Pirozzi T, et al. Cutoff score on the apathy evaluation scale in subjects with traumatic brain injury. Brain Inj 2002;16:509–16.
16. Starkstein SE, Mayberg HS, Preziosi TJ, et al. Reliability, validity, and clinical correlates of apathy in Parkinson's disease. J Neuropsychiatry Clin Neurosci 1992;4:134–9.
17. Strauss ME, Sperry SD. An informant-based assessment of apathy in Alzheimer disease. Neuropsychiatry Neuropsychol Behav Neurol 2002;15:176–83.
18. Robert PH, Clairet S, Benoit M, et al. The apathy inventory: assessment of apathy and awareness in Alzheimer's disease, Parkinson's disease and mild cognitive impairment. Int J Geriatr Psychiatry 2002;17:1099–105.
19. Sockeel P, Dujardin K, Devos D, et al. The Lille apathy rating scale (LARS), a new instrument for detecting and quantifying apathy: validation in Parkinson's disease. J Neurol Neurosurg Psychiatr 2006;77:579–84.
20. Grace J, Stout JC, Malloy PF. Assessing frontal lobe behavioral syndromes with the frontal lobe personality scale. Assessment 1999;6:269–84.
21. Niemeier JP, Perrin PB, Holcomb MG, et al. Factor structure, reliability, and validity of the Frontal Systems Behavior Scale (FrSBe) in an acute traumatic brain injury population. Rehabil Psychol 2013;58:51–63.
22. Cummings JL. The neuropsychiatric inventory: assessing psychopathology in dementia patients. Neurology 1997;48(Suppl 6):S10–6.
23. Lane-Brown A, Tate R. Interventions for apathy after traumatic brain injury. Cochrane Database Syst Rev 2009;(2):CD006341.
24. Muller U, Czymmek J, Thone-Otto A, et al. Reduced daytime activity in patients with acquired brain damage and apathy: a study with ambulatory actigraphy. Brain Inj 2006;20:157–60.

25. Ribot TH. Les malades de la volonte. 18th edition. Paris: Alcan; 1904.
26. Marin RS. Differential diagnosis and classification of apathy. Am J Psychiatry 1990;147:22–30.
27. Starkstein SE, Berthier M, Leiguarda R. Psychic akinesia following bilateral pallidal lesions. Int J Psychiatry Med 1989;19:155–64.
28. Laplane D, Dubois B. Auto-activation deficit: a basal ganglia related syndrome. Mov Disord 2001;16:810–4.
29. Habib M. Athymhormia and disorders of motivation in basal ganglia disease. J Neuropsychiatry Clin Neurosci 2004;16:509–24.
30. Al-Adawi S, Dorvlo AS, Burke DT, et al. Apathy and depression in cross-cultural survivors of traumatic brain injury. J Neuropsychiatry Clin Neurosci 2004;16:435–42.
31. Lane-Brown AT, Tate RL. Measuring apathy after traumatic brain injury: psychometric properties of the apathy evaluation scale and the frontal systems behavior scale. Brain Inj 2009;23:999–1007.
32. van Reekum R, Stuss DT, Ostrander L. Apathy: why care? J Neuropsychiatry Clin Neurosci 2005;17:7–19.
33. Ciurli P, Formisano R, Bivona U, et al. Neuropsychiatric disorders in persons with severe traumatic brain injury: prevalence, phenomenology, and relationship with demographic, clinical, and functional features. J Head Trauma Rehabil 2011;26:116–26.
34. Starkstein SE, Merello M, Jorge R, et al. The syndromal validity and nosological position of apathy in Parkinson's disease. Mov Disord 2009;24:1211–6.
35. Starkstein SE, Fedoroff JP, Price TR, et al. Apathy following cerebrovascular lesions. Stroke 1993;24:1625–30.
36. Starkstein SE. Apathy and withdrawal. Int Psychogeriatr 2000;12:135–8.
37. Andersson S, Krogstad JM, Finset A. Apathy and depressed mood in acquired brain damage: relationship to lesion localization and psychophysiological reactivity. Psychol Med 1999;29:447–56.
38. Starkstein SE, Merello M. Psychiatric and cognitive disorders in Parkinson's disease. Cambridge (MA): Cambridge University Press; 2002.
39. Andersson S, Bergedalen AM. Cognitive correlates of apathy in traumatic brain injury. Neuropsychiatry Neuropsychol Behav Neurol 2002;15:184–91.
40. Rao V, McCann U, Bergey A, et al. Correlates of apathy during the first year after traumatic brain injury. Psychosomatics 2013;54:403–4.
41. Paradiso S, Chemerinski E, Yazici KM, et al. Frontal lobe syndrome reassessed: comparison of patients with lateral or medial frontal brain damage. J Neurol Neurosurg Psychiatr 1999;67:664–7.
42. Finset A, Andersson S. Coping strategies in patients with acquired brain injury: relationships between coping, apathy, depression and lesion location. Brain Inj 2000;14:887–905.
43. Knutson KM, Monte OD, Raymont V, et al. Neural correlates of apathy revealed by lesion mapping in participants with traumatic brain injuries. Hum Brain Mapp 2013. [Epub ahead of print].
44. Spalletta G, Fagioli S, Caltagirone C, et al. Brain microstructure of subclinical apathy phenomenology in healthy individuals. Hum Brain Mapp 2013;34:3193–203.
45. Goldfine AM, Schiff ND. What is the role of brain mechanisms underlying arousal in recovery of motor function after structural brain injuries? Curr Opin Neurol 2011;24:564–9.
46. Newburn G, Newburn D. Selegiline in the management of apathy following traumatic brain injury. Brain Inj 2005;19:149–54.

47. Van Reekum R, Bayley M, Garner S, et al. N of 1 study: amantadine for the amotivational syndrome in a patient with traumatic brain injury. Brain Inj 1995;9: 49–53.
48. Tenovuo O. Central acetylcholinesterase inhibitors in the treatment of chronic traumatic brain injury - clinical experience in 111 patients. Prog Neuropsychopharmacol Biol Psychiatry 2005;1:61–7.
49. Muller U, Von Cramon DY. The therapeutic potential of bromocriptine in neuropsychological rehabilitation of patients with acquired brain damage. Prog Neuropsychopharmacol Biol Psychiatry 1994;18:1103–20.
50. Gualtieri CT, Evans RW. Stimulant treatment for the neurobehavioural sequelae of traumatic brain injury. Brain Inj 1988;2:273–90.
51. Smith RB, Tiberi A, Marshall J. The use of cranial electrotherapy stimulation in the treatment of closed-head-injured patients. Brain Inj 1994;8:357–61.

Psychotic Disorder Caused by Traumatic Brain Injury

Daryl E. Fujii, PhD[a],*, Iqbal Ahmed, MD[b,c]

KEYWORDS

- Psychosis • Mental disorder • Brain • Trauma

KEY POINTS

- Delusional disorders and schizophrenia-like psychoses are the most common psychotic syndromes among persons with traumatic brain injury (TBI); the former includes Capgras syndrome (ie, the delusion that loved ones are replaced by identical impostors) and reduplicative paramnesias (ie, delusions that places and buildings are replications of the real thing that are moved elsewhere), whereas schizophrenia-like psychosis includes persecutory delusions and auditory hallucinations.
- Delusional disorders tend to develop during the first year after injury, whereas schizophrenia-like psychoses are generally of delayed onset (ie, 3 to 4 years after injury).
- Psychotic disorders after TBI are often associated with focal lesions on magnetic resonance imaging/computed tomography in the frontal and temporal lobes, slowing in these regions on electroencephalogram, and cognitive impairments (ie, memory and executive function deficits).
- Psychosis among persons with TBI usually requires treatment with antipsychotics; anticonvulsants also may be useful. Emotional lability, irritability, impulsivity, or aggression are prominent concurrent symptoms.

Psychosis is a rare but severe sequela of TBI. Early studies with primarily open head injury cases from World War II and less standardized criteria for psychosis reported prevalence rates between 0.07% and 9.8%.[1] More contemporary studies with better methodologies consisting primarily of closed head injuries report rates in approximately the same range, from 0.9% to 8.5%.[2–7]

We would like to acknowledge Daniel Fujii for his assistance in procuring and reanalyzing data from previous papers and in performing some of the writing of the manuscript.
Funding Sources: None.
Conflict of Interest: None.
Disclaimer: The views expressed in this publication/presentation are those of the author(s) and do not reflect the official policy or position of the Department of the Army, Department of Defense, or the US Government.
[a] Veterans Affairs Pacific Island Health Care Services, Community Living Center, 459 Patterson Road, Honolulu, HI 96819, USA; [b] Department of Psychiatry, Tripler Army Medical Center, University of Hawaii, 1 Jarrett White Road, Honolulu, HI 96859, USA; [c] Uniformed Services University, 4301 Jones Bridge Road, Bethesda, MD 20814, USA
* Corresponding author.
E-mail address: dfujii07@gmail.com

Psychiatr Clin N Am 37 (2014) 113–124
http://dx.doi.org/10.1016/j.psc.2013.11.006
0193-953X/14/$ – see front matter Published by Elsevier Inc.

psych.theclinics.com

Abbreviations	
CT	Computed tomography
DD	Delusional disorder
DSM-5	Diagnostic and Statistical Manual of Mental Disorders, fifth edition
MRI	Magnetic resonance imaging
PDDTBI	Psychotic disorder caused by another medical condition: traumatic brain injury
PET	Positron emission tomography
PORT	Schizophrenia Patient Outcomes Research Team
PTSD	Posttraumatic stress disorder
SLP	Schizophrenia-like psychosis
TBI	Traumatic brain injury

According to DSM-5 nomenclature,[8] psychosis caused by a TBI is in the diagnostic category of PDDTBI. This diagnosis requires the presence of prominent hallucinations or delusions that are direct physiologic consequences of TBI, and not better accounted for by another mental disorder or delirium, and cause clinically significant distress or impairment in social, occupational, or other important areas of everyday function. When this condition develops, it may become chronic. Although the DSM-5 leaves uncertainty with regard to the specific features of this condition, the manual suggests that features suggesting PDDTBI may include a temporal association between medical condition and onset of psychosis; atypical features of psychosis, such as late age of onset or visual or olfactory hallucinations; occurrence in younger age groups; preexisting cognitive impairments as well as visual and hearing impairments, which may be risk factors with possible mechanisms lowering the threshold for experiencing a psychosis; and a lack of personal or family history of schizophrenia or DD.[8]

Accurate diagnosis of PDDTBI is important to both clinicians and researchers. From a clinical perspective, diagnosis guides treatment and informs prognosis. An accurate differential is also pertinent within a medicolegal context, in which compensation for damages from TBI are based on determining whether there is a preponderance of evidence that TBI caused a psychosis versus another disorder, most likely schizophrenia. From a research perspective, the study of PDDTBI may advance understanding of not only this condition but also of psychotic disorders more generally.

This article assists clinicians in diagnosing PDDTBI, by describing pertinent literature for each criterion and providing recommendations for treating the disorder. The data on which this article is predicated are derived from case series and observational studies published in the peer-reviewed literature over the last 30 years.[9,10] Informed by these reports, it first describes the presentation of PDDTBI as occurring in 2 general subtypes: DDs and SLP. The history and laboratory findings that support TBI as a causative factor in the development of a psychosis are discussed, and the need to differentiate PDDTBI from other psychotic disorders as well as delirium is highlighted. Treatments for PDDTBI, including psychopharmacologic and nonpharmacologic interventions, then are reviewed. In addition, a theoretic model of psychosis as a neurobehavioral syndrome and the proposed relationships between TBI and psychosis are presented for consideration and future study.

DIAGNOSIS OF PSYCHOSIS CAUSED BY TBI
Psychotic Symptoms

There are 2 general categories of PDDTBI: DDs and SLP. DD involves the occurrence of delusions only. According to analyses of case studies in the literature (n = 19),[9,10] the most common DDs are Capgras syndrome (ie, the delusion that loved ones are replaced by identical impostors) and reduplicative paramnesia (ie, the delusion that a familiar place such as home is duplicated in another location), each of which occurs with a frequency of approximately 32%. Other common delusions in this population include delusional jealousy (16%), Cotard syndrome (ie, the delusion of being dead or dying; 16%), somatic delusions (11%), and Fregoli (ie, the delusion of doubles, in which the person believes that different people are a single person who changes in appearance or who is in disguise; 5%). In contrast with primary psychotic disorders (ie, schizophrenia), negative symptoms are uncommon, occurring in only 25% of cases.

SLP caused by TBI typically involves the occurrence of hallucinations and delusions. Across published studies of this condition (n = 71),[9,10] the most common symptoms are hallucinations (97%), with 88% of cases presenting with auditory hallucinations and 22% with visual hallucinations. Delusions also are present in 85% of cases. The most common type of delusion is persecutory (65%); bizarre delusions, ideas of reference, and grandiose delusions occur less often (20%, 18%, and 16%, respectively). Negative symptoms are present in only 43% of PDDTBI; such features in the subgroup with negative symptoms include blunted affect (70%), social withdrawal (49%), and poor hygiene (40%). The general pattern of persecutory delusions, auditory hallucinations, and less prominent negative symptoms is a consistent finding in the literature.[1,5,11,12]

Relationship of Psychosis to TBI

Establishing that psychotic symptoms are the direct physiologic consequences of TBI is challenging. The strongest evidence for TBI as a cause of psychosis is the absence of psychotic symptoms or prodromal symptoms before the onset of TBI combined with the abrupt onset of psychotic symptoms within months after the TBI. However, the literature indicates that for many there is a delayed onset of psychosis after sustaining a TBI. For DD caused by TBI, in 64% of cases the onset of symptoms was less than a year after sustaining a TBI, whereas the overall mean latency between TBI and onset of psychosis was 3.3 years. For patients who developed an SLP after TBI, 42% showed psychotic symptoms within a year, 53% within 2 years, 63% within 3 years, and 72% before 4 years, with a mean delay of 3.3 years after the injury. Other studies report a similar pattern, with mean latencies between injury and psychosis onset of 4 to 5 years.[9,12,13] Prodromal symptoms are not universally present, but one study[12] evaluating them suggests that most persons developing an SLP after TBI do have behavioral changes that antedate frank psychosis, including bizarre behavior (50%), affective instability (39%), antisocial behavior (36%), scholastic or work deterioration (33%), and social withdrawal (31%).

Findings from neurologic studies and neuropsychological test data from case studies in the literature are presented in **Table 1**. For DD, 94% showed positive findings on MRI/CT with the most common lesions located in the frontal (75%) and temporal (56%) areas, followed by enlarged ventricles (38%). On electroencephalogram (EEG) studies, 71% showed positive findings. Of these, 43% reported slowing and 14% spiking, with common localization to temporal (29%) and frontal (14%) areas. All DD cases showed deficits on neuropsychological testing with impairments in memory (73%) and executive functioning (55%) the most common.

Among persons with SLP, functional neuroimaging seems to be more revealing of clinically relevant abnormalities than structural neuroimaging. All cases showed findings on single-photon emission CT (SPECT)/PET with most localized to temporal areas (86%). Eighty-seven percent of SLP cases reported positive findings on EEG with slowing (69%) and spiking (27%) the most common abnormality with localization to

Table 1 Laboratory findings associated with DD and SLP caused by TBI		
	DD	SLP
MRI/CT: positive findings (%)	94	55
Most common finding (%)	75 frontal 56 temporal 38 enlarged ventricles	34 frontal 19 temporal 19 enlarged ventricles
SPECT/PET: positive findings (%)	— — —	100 86 temporal 14 frontal
EEG: positive findings (%)	71	87
Most common finding (%)	29 temporal 14 frontal 43 slowing 14 spiking	53 temporal 23 frontal 69 slowing 27 spiking
Neuropsychological testing (%)	100 deficits	100 deficits
Most common finding (%)	73 memory 55 executive functioning	85 memory 65 executive functioning

Abbreviations: EEG, electroencephalogram; SPECT, single-photon emission computed tomography.

temporal (53%) and frontal (23%) areas. By contrast, roughly half of the SLP cases reported positive findings on MRI/CT (55%). Similar to DD, although at a much lower frequency, the most common areas of localization were frontal (34%) and temporal (19%) areas, and enlarged ventricles (19%). All SLP cases showed deficits on neuropsychological testing with memory (85%) and executive functioning (65%) the most common deficits. The preponderance of frontal and temporal findings on imaging studies is consistent with the literature.[1,5,11,12]

There does not seem to be a strong dose-dependent relationship between severity of TBI and onset of psychosis, because psychosis can result from both mild and moderate to severe injuries.[6,7,9,11–16] For cases in the literature that developed a DD after TBI, 82% sustained a loss of consciousness, with 29% deemed to have sustained a mild TBI and 71% moderate to severe according to criteria set by the Mild Traumatic Brain Injury Committee of the Head Injury Interdisciplinary Special Interest Group of the American Congress of Rehabilitation Medicine.[17] In a similar way, 82% of SLP cases sustained a loss of consciousness, with 44% showing a mild TBI and 56% a TBI in the moderate to severe range.

The observation that a psychotic disorder may follow a mild TBI is consistent with the possibility of vulnerability factors that increase risk for psychosis after any injury type or severity. Such risk factors include family history of psychotic illness and prior neurologic or neurodevelopmental conditions.[9,10,12] For example, in the combined case studies in the PDDTBI literature, for cases that developed a DD, 44% sustained a seizure disorder, whereas 25% had a family history of mental illness. For those developing SLP, 38% reported a comorbid seizure disorder, and 38% had a family history of mental illness. Thus, mild TBI might be more likely to produce psychosis in an individual at increased risk for this condition because of premorbid risk factors or postinjury seizure disorder.

Differential Diagnosis

The principal alternatives to PDDTBI are primary psychotic disorders (eg, schizophrenia, schizoaffective disorder, DD), substance-induced psychotic disorder, psychotic disorder caused by another medical condition (eg, seizure disorder), and PTSD. Differentiating PDDTBI from schizophrenia can be difficult because of the overlap in presentation, risk factors, and neuropathology. Both are characterized by delusions, auditory hallucinations, and a pattern of neuropsychological deficits with most salient impairments in executive functioning and memory.[8] Family history of psychotic disorder is a strong risk factor for both disorders.[18] Frontal and temporal lobe lesions are also common findings on neuroimaging studies.[19] Adding to the differential complexity, patients with schizophrenia may also have an increased risk for head trauma.[20]

Despite the similarities, there seem to be several distinguishing features (**Table 2**). Persons with PDDTBI seem to exhibit fewer negative symptoms than persons with schizophrenia.[10] On structural neuroimaging studies, PDDTBI is associated with more focal lesions to temporal and frontal lobes versus schizophrenia, which is associated with enlarged ventricles and generalized atrophy including temporal lobes, particularly the hippocampus, frontal lobes, and subcortical structures including the thalamus and basal ganglia.[21] On functional neuroimaging, PDDTBI is associated with both temporal and frontal findings, whereas schizophrenia is associated with abnormal activity in several areas, including frontal lobes, temporal lobes, basal ganglia, and thalamus.[10,21] In addition, on EEG the most common finding for PDDTBI is temporal spiking compared with normal EEG or occasional increased presence of slow waves, particularly in the frontal regions found in schizophrenia.[22]

Substance-induced psychotic disorders and PDDTBI also are challenging to differentiate from one another, especially among persons with substance use disorders after TBI. Individuals who abuse substances are at higher risk to sustain a TBI, including severe TBI.[23] Increased baseline behavioral tendencies toward impulsivity and risk taking increase the risk for substance abuse and TBI.[24] Severe preinjury substance abuse may cause psychotic symptoms and new or continued postinjury substance use may do so as well. These facts may collectively interact such that premorbid vulnerabilities (manifest as behaviors like impulsivity and risk taking) increase the risk of substance use

Table 2
Potential characteristics that discriminate between PDDTBI and schizophrenia

	PDDTBI	Schizophrenia
Presence of negative symptoms (%)	43 70 blunted affect 40 social withdrawal 40 disheveled	50–90[44] 46 social withdrawal 33 blunted affect[45] —
MRI/CT: positive findings (%)	55	12–35[46–49]
Atrophy (%)	0	12–35[50,51]
Focal abnormalities (%)	89	6–9[52,53]
Most common finding (%)	34 frontal 19 temporal 19 enlarged ventricles	Frontal, temporal Hippocampal, basal Ganglia, thalamus atrophy, enlarged ventricles[21]
SPECT/PET: positive findings (%)	100 86 temporal 14 frontal	Frontal, temporal, thalamus Basal ganglia hypoperfusion 20–60[54]
EEG: positive findings (%)	87	—
Most common finding (%)	60 slowing 53 temporal	Frontal slowing[22]

and TBI and may interact to increase the risk of psychosis. As an aid to differential diagnosis, psychotic symptoms tend to be time limited if they are entirely caused by substance abuse.[8] However, chronic use of dopaminergic agonists such as methamphetamine, cocaine, or marijuana can also result in a psychosis that persists and may increase risk for such among persons with TBI even when substance use ceases.[25]

Psychosis caused by seizure disorder also is challenging to distinguish from PDDTBI and, in some cases, these conditions may co-occur. However, it is important to attempt to determine whether one or both of these conditions are present because these diagnoses entail different treatments. The percentage of seizure-related psychosis in our combined PDDTBI case studies[9,10] is 32%. However, 84% of patients showed positive findings on EEG, with 53% occurring in the temporal lobes. This finding suggests the possibility that, like persons in the general population,[26] symptomatically important simple or complex partial seizures may be under-recognized in persons with PDDTBI.[26]

Partial complex seizures, especially those originating from the temporal lobes, may lead to psychotic symptoms that can be ictal, postictal, or interictal in nature. Ictal and postictal psychoses tend to be episodic and occur in close temporal relationship to a seizure; attributing psychoses of these types to seizures therefore is straightforward. Even among persons with TBI, the occurrence of psychosis in close temporal proximity to a seizure and an EEG showing epileptiform discharges strongly suggests epilepsy as the best explanation for psychosis. In such cases, treatment is directed principally at the epilepsy rather than at psychosis alone. However, distinguishing interictal psychosis from SLP-type PDDTBI is more challenging, because the temporal relationship between psychosis onset and either seizures or TBI is variable, their phenomenologies are similar, and both may become chronic problems.[27] In such cases, clear attribution of the psychosis to epilepsy or TBI may not be possible and concurrent treatments targeting both epilepsy and psychotic symptoms may be required.

With the large numbers of soldiers returning from the wars in Iraq and Afghanistan with PTSD and blast head injuries, clinicians may experience some difficulty distinguishing severe intrusion and dissociative symptoms caused by PTSD from symptoms of PDDTBI. Although not a psychotic disorder, severe PTSD may be associated with auditory and visual hallucinations as well as persecutory delusions. However, symptoms tend to be specific to the traumatic event or war experiences and can become chronic.[28] Hallucinations or delusions that are not war related are more likely to suggest PDDTBI.

Delirium also is in the differential diagnosis of PDDTBI, and refers to a state of altered attention and fluctuating sensorium with attendant cognitive, behavioral, physical symptoms.[8] When delirium caused by TBI develops, it is a feature of the immediate postinjury period (especially following moderate or severe TBI) and is a transient phenomenon (albeit one that may persist for days or weeks following TBI). Psychotic symptoms, particularly visual hallucinations, occurring during this period are best explained as symptoms of delirium. PDDTBI psychotic symptoms must occur in the context of a clear sensorium and are typically characterized by auditory hallucinations and delusions.[29]

Functional Consequences of PDDTBI

The DSM-5 specifies that PDDTBI involves symptoms that cause clinically significant distress or impairment in social, occupational, or other important areas of functioning. The addition of this criterion to the DSM-5 set describing psychoses caused by another medical condition is new and reflects the trend toward reserving clinical diagnosis for symptoms that are subjectively or functionally relevant. Psychotic symptoms that do not significantly disrupt the person's life are therefore not considered to meet criteria for PDDTBI.

TREATMENT
Pharmacotherapy

Pharmacologic treatment of PDDTBI is similar in many respects to the treatment of schizophrenia or other DDs. Most persons with PDDTBI receive treatment with antipsychotics and require only 1 medication for this condition. The literature describing the pharmacotherapy for PDD does not show the superiority of any particular antipsychotic or class of antipsychotics for this purpose, and clinician judgment dictates their prescription. Some persons with PDDTBI require concurrent treatment with additional medications, including anticonvulsants and/or antidepressants. Individual symptoms and their response to these agents inform the pharmacotherapy for PDDTBI, which again parallels the approach to the treatment of symptoms associated with primary psychotic disorders.

Patients with PDDTBI are more susceptible to adverse effects such as increased sedation, anticholinergic effects, and extrapyramidal syndromes than even patients with primary psychiatric disorders. Especially in the weeks and months after the TBI, issues such as high comorbidity with seizure disorder, a lowered seizure threshold caused by the TBI, and the potential effect of delaying neuronal recovery after TBI are additional considerations.[30] Because of the high comorbidity with secondary seizure disorders or underlying seizure diathesis, differences in seizure risk from antipsychotics or other psychotropics should be a considered when selecting a medication.[31,32] A viable option is to trial anticonvulsants before prescribing antipsychotics, especially if mood lability, impulsivity, irritability, or affective aggression are salient symptoms.[30]

Clinicians also need to remain mindful of the potential adverse effects of antipsychotics on neuronal recovery in the early weeks after a TBI.[30] The principle of starting low, and going slow, but staying the course should be followed when prescribing antipsychotics. Ongoing assessment for continued need for medications should be conducted to reduce the risk of long-term adverse effects from antipsychotics, including tardive dyskinesia and metabolic syndrome. Treatment of other sequelae such as cognitive symptoms, sleep, mood disorders, and substance abuse that may coexist with the psychosis should be targeted to facilitate coping and improve psychotic symptoms.

Nonpharmacologic Treatment

Although not specifically developed for, or validated on, the PDDTBI population, evidence-based psychosocial treatments for persons with schizophrenia may be useful to address impairments in social and vocational functioning.[33] These approaches to treatment are essential components of the management of psychotic disorders in general, and seem to benefit negative symptoms, cognitive deficits, and family dynamics as well.[33] The PORT psychosocial treatment recommendations[33] suggest that psychosocial interventions for persons with schizophrenia include assertive community training, supported employment, cognitive behavior therapy, family-based services, token economy, skills training, psychosocial interventions for alcohol and substance use disorders, and psychosocial interventions for weight management. Other emerging interventions for this population focus on medication adherence and cognitive remediation, as well as peer support and peer-delivered services. Use of these interventions with persons with PDDTBI has not been studied systematically and their adaptation (especially for cognitive impairments and co-occurring physical impairments and medication conditions) may be required in order for them to be useful in persons with TBI. Nonetheless, the PORT treatment recommendations and summary may be useful for clinicians working with persons with PDDTBI to consider.

THEORETIC MODEL OF THE PROPOSED RELATIONSHIPS BETWEEN TBI AND PSYCHOSIS

Given the similarities in the presentation and localization of cerebral lesions on neuroimaging studies across psychotic conditions with different causes, Fujii and Ahmed[15] (2004) argued that psychosis is a neurobehavioral disorder similar to aphasia and apraxia. In neurobehavioral disorders, damage to components of the associated neurocircuit, regardless of cause, result in similar behaviors. For example, lesions to Wernicke's area produce a fluent aphasia. Nonfluent aphasias are associated with lesions to the Broca's area, and conduction aphasia results from lesions to the arcuate fasciculus. Despite similarities in presentation, qualitative differences may exist caused by severity and location of damage within the system, specific mechanism of damage, and severity and amount of damage.

Fujii and Ahmed[34] (2007) therefore proposed criteria for a behavioral syndrome disorder to be considered a neurobehavioral disorder. Each criterion will be followed by supportive evidence from the PDDTBI literature as well as findings from other secondary psychoses. First, a constellation of symptoms is reliably associated with neuropathology in a circumscribed structural location or neural circuit. Delusions and auditory hallucinations in schizophrenia are associated with neuropathology in the frontal and temporal-hippocampal areas.[35,36] These observations inform the phenomenology and neurobiology of PDDTBI.

Second, disturbances in specific neural circuits or localized lesions secondary to different etiologies will present with similar behavioral or cognitive symptoms. Persecutory delusions and auditory hallucinations in PDDTBI closely align with common positive symptoms in schizophrenia. The most common findings on imaging studies in PDDTBI are lesions to frontal and temporal areas.[1,5,9,11,12,16] The onset and symptom development in PDDTBI and schizophrenia are also similar. During the early stages of schizophrenia, patients experience a functional decline and show psychiatric symptoms before onset of the full-fledged psychotic disorder. The duration of prodromes is highly variable, with a bimodal distribution ranging from less than a year to 4.5 years.[37] Findings in PDDTBI research also report a bimodal latency period between the TBI and the onset of psychosis. In one study, all cases of PPDTBI were preceded by a prodrome.[12]

Third, in general, smaller amounts of similar neurobiological disturbances are associated with milder symptoms. PDDTBI is associated with more focal lesions, whereas schizophrenia is associated with global atrophy. Schizophrenia is associated with more severe functional impairments, as shown by a greater likelihood of negative symptoms[9,12] and more severe cognitive impairment[15] that are strongly associated with illness severity and long-term prognosis.[38–41]

Fourth, additional symptoms such as cognitive, mood, psychiatric, or other associated neurologic symptoms are related to other networks simultaneously being affected by underlying neurochemical or neuropathologic processes. Lesions to frontal (PET) and temporal (CT/MRI) areas in schizophrenia have been reliably correlated with cognitive impairments in executive functioning and memory, the two most common neuropsychological deficits in schizophrenia.[42] In PDDTBI, frontal and temporal abnormalities[1,5,9,11,12,16] and impairments in executive functioning and memory[9,10,12,15] are robust findings.

Fifth, aside from treating the underlying disease process, treatment of the associated symptoms of a neurobiological disorder of different causes is similar. The

PDDTBI literature reports that antipsychotics are the most commonly prescribed and efficacious medications for treating positive symptoms of the disorder.[9,12]

Within this conceptual framework for psychosis as a neurobehavioral syndrome, we propose the following possible relationships between TBI and psychosis:

1. TBI may contribute to the development of a psychosis by expediting the onset of a psychosis in someone who is at high risk and would have converted to psychosis in the future (eg, a person with a genetic predisposition who is showing significant prodromal symptoms such as attenuated positive symptoms); causing the cumulative amount of damage to the brain circuits involved in psychotic symptoms to surpass the threshold needed for the onset of a psychosis in a person who would not otherwise have experienced psychotic symptoms (eg, a person with previous TBI or genetic predisposition without prodromal symptoms); triggering a process of neurologic or neurochemical changes that induces secondary epilepsy that results in a psychosis; and/or damaging frontal systems and reducing normal inhibitory controls over behaviors. The individual then engages in risky behaviors that result in further brain damage to surpass the threshold to develop a psychosis (eg, a person starts abusing substances such as methamphetamine or cocaine or engages in risky behaviors that result in additional brain injuries).
2. TBI can exacerbate the symptoms and severity of an existing psychosis by worsening the extent of damage to circuits associated with psychosis; and/or worsening coping skills, thus leading to dysregulation of stress hormones and neurotransmitters such as glutamate and dopamine (a review of relationship between stress and psychotic symptoms in schizophrenia is given by Myin-Germeys[43]).
3. TBI can increase vulnerability to developing a psychosis by increasing biologic vulnerability so that future damage or changes to frontal or temporal structures, and the underlying neurotransmitter systems (eg, damage sustained through trauma, disease, substance abuse, neuronal and biochemical changes during normal human development), trigger a psychosis, inducing physiologic and psychological changes that render the individual more vulnerable to stress, and thereby leading to dysregulation of stress hormones and neurotransmitters such as glutamate and dopamine in an individual with compromised regulation of dopamine (eg, frontal dysregulation, physical disabilities, pain).
4. TBI may be unrelated to the development of psychosis.

SUMMARY AND FUTURE DIRECTIONS

PDDTBI is an uncommon but serious neurobehavioral disorder. It has 2 major subtypes: DDs and SLP, the phenomenologies of which are similar to their idiopathic counterparts except for negative symptoms, which are less common among persons with PDDTBI. The similarities between PDDTBI and other psychotic disorders, including their phenomenology, risk factors, and neuropathology, make differentiating between them challenging. The conceptual framework of psychosis as a neurobehavioral syndrome presented here encourages approaching the development of psychosis after TBI from the perspective of the effects of injury on frontal and temporal circuits and the interaction between injury and vulnerability factors for psychosis. Evaluation informed by this approach may facilitate characterization of the relationship between TBI and psychosis in an individual patient and inform the pharmacotherapies and psychosocial interventions used to reduce the symptoms of psychosis as well as their adverse effects on subjective well-being and everyday function.

REFERENCES

1. Davison K, Bagley CR. Schizophrenia-like psychoses associated with organic disorders of the central nervous system: a review of the literature. Br J Psychiatry Suppl 1969;114:113–62.
2. Chen YH, Chiu WT, Chu SF, et al. Increased risk of schizophrenia following traumatic brain injury: a 5-year follow-up study in Taiwan. Psychol Med 2011;41(6): 1271–7.
3. Fann JR, Leonetti A, Jaffe K, et al. Psychiatric illness and subsequent traumatic brain injury: a case control study. J Neurol Neurosurg Psychiatry 2002;72: 615–20.
4. Silver JM, Kramer R, Greenwald S, et al. The association between head injuries and psychiatric disorders: findings from the New Haven NIMH epidemiological catchment area study. Brain Inj 2001;15:935–45.
5. Violin A, De Mol J. Psychological sequelae after head traumas in adults. Acta Neurochir (Wien) 1987;85:96–102.
6. Harrison G, Whitley E, Rasmussen F, et al. Risk of schizophrenia and other non-affective psychosis among individual exposed to head injury: case control study. Schizophr Res 2006;88:119–26.
7. Nielsen AS, Mortensen PB, O'Callaghan EO, et al. Is head injury a risk factor for schizophrenia? Schizophr Res 2002;55:93–8.
8. American Psychiatric Association. Diagnostic and statistical manual of mental disorders. 5th edition. Washington, DC: American Psychiatric Association; 2013.
9. Fujii DE, Ahmed I. Psychosis due to traumatic brain injury: an analysis of case studies in the literature. J Neuropsychiatry Clin Neurosci 2002;14:130–40.
10. Fujii DE, Fujii DC. Psychotic disorder due to traumatic brain injury: analysis of case studies in the literature. J Neuropsychiatry Clin Neurosci 2012;24: 278–89.
11. Achte KA, Hilllbom E, Aalberg V. Psychoses following war injuries. Acta Psychiatr Scand 1969;45:1–18.
12. Sachdev P, Smith JS, Cathcart S. Schizophrenia-like psychosis following traumatic brain injury: a chart-based descriptive and case-control study. Psychol Med 2001;31:231–9.
13. Fujii DE, Ahmed I. Risk factors in psychosis secondary to traumatic brain injury. J Neuropsychiatry Clin Neurosci 2001;13:61–9.
14. Fann JR, Burington B, Leonetti A, et al. Psychiatric illness following traumatic brain injury in an adult health maintenance organization population. Arch Gen Psychiatry 2004;61:53–61.
15. Fujii DE, Ahmed I, Hishinuma E. A neuropsychological comparison of psychotic disorder following traumatic brain injury, traumatic brain injury without psychotic disorder, and schizophrenia. J Neuropsychiatry Clin Neurosci 2004; 16:306–14.
16. Koponen S, Taiminen T, Portin R, et al. Axis I and II psychiatric disorders after traumatic brain injury: a 30-year follow-up study. Am J Psychiatry 2002;159: 1315–21.
17. Mild Traumatic Brain Injury Committee of the Head Injury Interdisciplinary Special Interest Group of the American Congress of Rehabilitation Medicine: definition of mild traumatic brain injury. J Head Trauma Rehabil 1993;8:86–7.
18. Kendler KS, McGuire M, Gruenberg AM, et al. An epidemiological, clinical, and family study of simple schizophrenia in County Roscommon, Ireland. Am J Psychiatry 1994;151:27–34.

19. Shepard AM, Laurens KR, Matheson SL, et al. Systematic meta-review and quality assessment of the structural brain alterations in schizophrenia. Neurosci Biobehav Rev 2012;36:1342–56.
20. Burg JS, McGuire LM, Burright RG, et al. Prevalence of traumatic brain injury in an inpatient psychiatric population. J Clin Psychol Med Settings 1996;3:245–51.
21. Ahmed AO, Buckley PF, Hanna M. Neuroimaging schizophrenia: a picture is worth a thousand words, but is it saying anything important? Curr Psychiatry Rep 2013;15:345.
22. Boutros NN, Arfken C, Galderisi S, et al. The status of spectral EEG abnormality as a diagnostic test for schizophrenia. Schizophr Res 2008;102:21–6.
23. Andelic N, Jerstad T, Sigurdardottir S, et al. Effects of acute substance abuse on traumatic brain injury severity in adults admitted to a trauma center. J Trauma Manag Outcomes 2010;4:6.
24. Bjork JM, Grant SJ. Does traumatic brain injury increase risk for substance abuse? J Neurotrauma 2009;26(7):1077–82.
25. Smith MJ, Thirthalli J, Abdallah AG, et al. Prevalence of psychotic symptoms in substance abusers: a comparison across substances. Compr Psychiatry 2009; 50:245–50.
26. Kotsopoulos IA, van Merode T, Kessels FG, et al. Systematic review and meta-analysis of incidence studies of epilepsy and unprovoked seizures. Epilepsia 2002;43(11):1402–9.
27. Elliott B, Joyce E, Shorvon S. Delusions, illusions and hallucinations in epilepsy: 2. Complex phenomena and psychosis. Epilepsy Res 2009;85:172–86.
28. Braakman MH, Kortman FA, van Den Brink W. Validity of 'post-traumatic stress disorder with secondary psychotic features': a review of the evidence. Acta Psychiatr Scand 2009;119:15–24.
29. Fujii D, Armstrong NP, Ahmed I. Psychotic disorder due to traumatic brain injury. In: Fujii D, Ahmed I, editors. The spectrum of psychotic disorders. Cambridge (United Kingdom): Cambridge University Press; 2007. p. 3–12.
30. Chew E, Zafonte RD. Pharmacological management of neurobehavioral disorders following traumatic brain injury–A state-of-the-art review. J Rehabil Res Dev 2009;46:851–78.
31. Alper K, Schwartz KA, Kolts RL, et al. Seizure incidence in psychopharmacological trials: an analysis of Food and Drug Administration (FDA) summary basis of approval reports. Biol Psychiatry 2007;62:345–54.
32. Kumlien E, Lundberg PO. Seizure risk associated with neuroactive drugs: data from the WHO adverse drug reactions database. Seizure 2010;19:69–73.
33. Dixon LB, Dickerson F, Bellack AS, et al. The 2009 schizophrenia PORT psychosocial treatment recommendations and summary statements. Schizophr Bull 2010;36:48–70.
34. Fujii D, Ahmed I. Is psychosis a neurobiological syndrome: integration and conclusion. In: Fujii D, Ahmed I, editors. The spectrum of psychotic disorders. Cambridge (United Kingdom): Cambridge University Press; 2007. p. 535–55.
35. Knobel A, Heinz A, Voss M. Imaging the deluded brain. Eur Arch Psychiatry Clin Neurosci 2008;258(Suppl 5):76–80.
36. Jardri R, Pouchet A, Pins D, et al. Cortical activations during auditory verbal hallucinations in schizophrenia: a coordinate-based meta-analysis. Am J Psychiatry 2011;168:73–81.
37. Yung AR, McGorry PD. The prodromal phase of first-episode psychosis: past and current conceptualizations. Schizophr Bull 1996;22:353–70.

38. White C, Stirling J, Hopkins R, et al. Predictors of 10-year outcome of first-episode psychosis. Psychol Med 2009;39:1447–56.
39. Hwu FG, Chen CH, Whang TJ, et al. Symptom patterns and subgrouping of schizophrenic patients: significant of negative symptoms assessed on admission. Schizophr Res 2002;56:105–19.
40. Fujii D, Wylie AM, Nathan JH. Neurocognition and long-term prediction of quality of life in outpatients with severe and persistent mental illness. Schizophr Res 2004;69:67–73.
41. Fujii DE, Wylie AM. Neurocognition and community outcome in schizophrenia: long-term predictive validity. Schizophr Res 2003;59:219–23.
42. Heinrichs RW, Zakzanis KK. Neurocognitive deficit in schizophrenia: a quantitative review of the evidence. Neuropsychology 1998;12:426–45.
43. Myin-Germeys I, van Os J. Stress-reactivity in psychosis: evidence for an affective pathway to psychosis. Clin Psychol Rev 2007;27:409–24.
44. Ritchie CE, Primelo R, Radke AQ. Bullet in the brain: a case of organic psychosis. J Neuropsychiatry Clin Neurosci 1989;1:449–51.
45. Morbidity and mortality weekly report. Incidence rates of hospitalization related to traumatic brain injury: 12 states, 2002. JAMA 2006;295(15):1764–5.
46. Ferguson PL, Smith GM, Wannamaker BB, et al. A population-based study of risk of epilepsy after hospitalization for traumatic brain injury. Epilepsia 2010; 51:891–8.
47. Makinen J, Miettunen J, Ishanni M, et al. Negative symptoms in schizophrenia: a review. Nord J Psychiatry 2008;62:334–41.
48. Bobes J, Arango C, Garci-Garcia M, et al. Prevalence of negative symptoms in outpatients with schizophrenia spectrum disorders treated with antipsychotics in routine clinical practice: findings from the CLAMORS study. J Clin Psychiatry 2010;71(3):280–6.
49. Breier A, Schrieber JL, Dyer J, et al. National Institute of Mental Health longitudinal study of chronic schizophrenia. Arch Gen Psychiatry 1991;48:239–46.
50. Cazzullo CL, Vita A, Sacchetti E, et al. Brain morphology in schizophrenic disorder: prevalence and correlates of diffuse (cortical and subcortical) brain atrophy. Psychiatry Res 1989;29:257–9.
51. Vita A, Sacchetti E, Calzeroni A, et al. Cortical atrophy in schizophrenia: prevalence and associated features. Schizophr Res 1988;1:329–37.
52. Nasrallah HA, Kuperman S, Hamra BJ, et al. Clinical differences between schizophrenic patients with and without large cerebral ventricles. J Clin Psychiatry 1983;44:407–10.
53. Vita A, Dieci M, Giobbio GM, et al. CT scan abnormalities and outcome in chronic schizophrenia. Am J Psychiatry 1991;148:1577–9.
54. Pearlson GD, Marsh L. Structural brain imaging in schizophrenia: a selective review. Biol Psychiatry 1999;46:627–49.

Neuropsychiatry of Pediatric Traumatic Brain Injury

Jeffrey E. Max, MBBCh

KEYWORDS

- Pediatric traumatic brain injury • Novel psychiatric disorder • Risk factors
- Treatment • Review • Brain imaging

KEY POINTS

- Pediatric traumatic brain injury (TBI) is a major public health problem.
- Psychiatric disorders with onset before the injury are more common than population base rates.
- Novel (postinjury onset) psychiatric disorders are also common and complicate child function after injury.
- Novel disorders include personality change due to TBI, secondary attention-deficit/hyperactivity disorder, other disruptive behavior disorders, and internalizing disorders.

INTRODUCTION

It is incumbent on health practitioners, including mental health practitioners, to be familiar with the neuropsychiatry of pediatric traumatic brain injury. This requirement is because of practical and theoretic concerns. The principal practical issue is related to the independent and overlapping public health significance of pediatric traumatic brain injury (TBI) and psychiatric disorders. The primary theoretic importance relates to understanding brain-behavior relationships within a developmental biopsychosocial model of psychiatric disorder.

EPIDEMIOLOGY

Pediatric TBI is a major public health problem with an annual incidence of 400 per 100,000, and is an important cause of death and disability in the United States.[1] The

Dr J.E. Max receives grant support from the National Institutes of Health (R-01 1R01HD068432-01A1). He provides expert testimony in cases of traumatic brain injury on an ad hoc basis for plaintiffs and defendants equally. This activity constitutes approximately 5% of his professional activity.
Neuropsychiatric Research, Rady Children's Hospital, 3020 Children's Way, MC 5018, San Diego, CA 92123-4282, USA
E-mail address: jmax@ucsd.edu

Psychiatr Clin N Am 37 (2014) 125–140
http://dx.doi.org/10.1016/j.psc.2013.11.003

Abbreviations	
ADHD	Attention-deficit/hyperactivity disorder
CAPS	Counselor-assisted problem solving
IRC	Internet resource comparison
NPD	Novel psychiatric disorders
NPRS	Neuropsychiatric Rating Schedule
ODD	Oppositional defiant disorder
PC	Personality change due to traumatic brain injury
PCIT	Parent-child interaction therapy
PTSD	Post-traumatic stress disorder
RUPPS	Research units in pediatric psychopharmacology
SADHD	Secondary attention-deficit/hyperactivity disorder
SPT	Single patient trial
SSRI	Selective serotonin reuptake inhibitor
TBI	Traumatic brain injury
TOPS	Teen online problem solving

male/female incidence rate ratio is approximately 1.8:1 and higher (2.2:1) in children aged 5 to 14 years. The incidence in boys and girls is similar in children aged 1 to 5 years (160 per 100,000 population), but then increases at a higher rate in boys. Brain injury rates increase for boys and decrease for girls in late childhood and adolescence. Higher incidence rates are significantly related to median family income even when age and/or race/ethnicity are controlled.[2] The proportion of brain injury caused by motor vehicle–related accidents increases with age from 20% in children 0 to 4 years old, up to 66% in adolescents.[3] Bicycle-related or pedestrian injuries are more likely to affect younger children, whereas injury in adolescents is more often linked to motor vehicle accidents. Mechanism of injury in almost half of cases of infant, toddler, and young child TBI is related to assaults or child abuse, and falls. The distribution of brain injury, by severity, ranges between 5% and 8% for severe, 7% and 8% for moderate, and 80% and 90% for mild brain injury.

PATHOPHYSIOLOGY

Focal injuries including intracerebral, subdural, and epidural hematomas occur with a lower incidence in children (15%–20%) versus adults (30%–42%). The frequency of focal lesions occurs in a rostrocaudal gradient. There is a higher frequency of children with lesions in the frontal lobe white matter, orbitofrontal region (orbital gyrus, gyrus rectus, and inferior frontal gyrus), and dorsolateral frontal region (middle and superior frontal gyri); a few lesions in the anterior temporal lobe; and isolated lesions in more posterior areas.[4] Skull fractures are evident in about 5% to 25% of children and are less commonly associated with epidural hematomas (40%) compared with adults (61%). Diffuse injury and cerebral swelling resulting in intracranial hypertension are more common in children than in adults. The principal neuropathologic findings of a diffuse injury in children are diffuse axonal injury and/or vascular injury. Reviews of advances and challenges in the understanding of the pathophysiology of pediatric TBI as well as initial assessment, management, and treatment of pediatric TBI are available.[5,6] Recognition and treatment of potential medical complications such as hypotension, hypoxemia, increased intracranial pressure, delirium, seizures, paresis, peripheral neuropathy, musculoskeletal problems, and endocrine disorders are important to decrease morbidity.

EVALUATION

The typical presentation of a child or adolescent with TBI to a mental health professional occurs at a variable amount of time after the injury. This requires a retrospective accounting of preinjury status and postinjury course of the presenting psychiatric syndrome. Asarnow and colleagues[7] provided a useful template for thinking about determinates of behavioral syndromes in children and adolescents with TBI. The pathways to behavioral issues include the following possibilities: (1) the behavior problem antedates the injury and may contribute to the risk for incurring the injury; (2) a preexisting behavior problem is exacerbated by the brain injury; (3) the behavior problem is a direct (biological) effect of a brain injury; (4) the behavior problem is an immediate secondary effect of the injury (eg, an emotional response to the accident, such as posttraumatic stress disorder [PTSD]); (5) the behavior problem is a long-term secondary effect of the injury (eg, the conduct problems and decreased motivation from frustration produced by the cognitive impairments caused by brain injury); (6) the behavior problems are caused by factors other than the injury.

The ability of clinicians to make rational decisions in cases of pediatric TBI is enhanced by familiarity with the relevant scientific database on psychiatric disorders and their risk factors. This article deals sequentially with methodological considerations, preinjury psychiatric status, and new-onset (postinjury) psychiatric disorders.

Methodological Concerns

There are only 4 published prospective studies of consecutive hospital admissions of children and adolescents with TBI in which standardized psychiatric interviews were used to assess psychopathology,[8–11] and only 2 of these studies had injured control children.[8,11,12] This small literature is complemented by a larger corpus that addresses postinjury behavioral changes reported by parents and teachers, typically by questionnaires, which tend not to be specific for the generating of psychiatric diagnoses or psychiatric treatment plans.[13–17] With rare exceptions,[18] studies exclude children with a history of nonaccidental injury. Therefore this article refers only to accidental injury.

Preinjury Psychiatric Status

Prospective psychiatric TBI studies that have used standardized psychiatric interviews found that between one-third and one-half of children had a preinjury lifetime psychiatric disorder.[8–11] The finding that children who have a TBI are on average more behaviorally affected before their injuries is supported by epidemiologic data from a birth cohort with data points at age 5 years and at age 10 years.[19] Children who went on to sustain injuries (including mild TBI, lacerations, and burns) between age 5 and 10 years had more behavioral problems, particularly aggression, before their injuries compared with uninjured children. One explanation for these findings involves a higher risk of injury in children with high impulsivity and risk-taking behaviors corresponding with diagnoses of externalizing disorders such as attention-deficit/hyperactivity disorder (ADHD)[20] in the absence of known preinjury brain damage.

Postinjury Psychiatric Status

The term novel psychiatric disorder (NPD) refers to 2 possible scenarios. In the first, a child who is free of preinjury lifetime psychiatric disorders may manifest a psychiatric disorder after injury. In the second, a child with a lifetime preinjury psychiatric disorder may develop a psychiatric disorder that was not present before the TBI. NPDs are heterogeneous; the forces related to each injury and the eventual precise patterns of brain damage are different in each case. The categorical classification (NPD vs no NPD) reflects functional outcome in children and informs clinicians about risk factors for psychiatric disorder in this population. However, research on the phenomenology and risk factors of specific NPDs or specific clusters of postinjury psychiatric symptoms is more useful both for the clinician who needs to tackle specific target symptoms and for the neuroscientist who seeks to understand brain-behavior relationships that may be applicable to both injured and noninjured children.

NPD

NPD recorded approximately 24 months after severe TBI has been present in 54% to 63% of children, and following mild/moderate TBI in 10% to 21% of children, and following orthopedic injury in 4% to 14% of children.[8,21,22] A recent study found that NPD was related to a lower fractional anisotropy in bilateral frontal and temporal lobes, bilateral centrum semiovale, and bilateral uncinate fasciculi.[12] In other studies, depending on time since injury, predictors of NPD have included severity of injury, preinjury psychiatric disorders, socioeconomic status/preinjury intellectual function, preinjury adaptive function, preinjury family function, and family psychiatric history.[8,22]

In recent years there has been a greater public awareness of pediatric mild TBI, and especially its overlap with sports concussion. Depending on study design, the rate of NPD in children with mild TBI varies from 10% to 100%.[8,21,23-26] However, in studies limited to consecutively treated children with mild TBI the range is narrower (10%–40%), with larger studies generally finding higher rates. The rate at which children with mild TBI versus injured controls developed NPD was similar in one study[8] and higher, although not significantly so, in other small underpowered studies.[21,27] In studies of TBI compared with uninjured controls, children with mild TBI had nonsignificantly higher,[28] marginally higher,[24] or significantly higher[23,29] rates of NPD in 4 studies. Studies suggest that children with mild/moderate or mild TBI were at significantly higher risk for developing new-onset psychiatric disorder or an increase in postconcussion symptoms respectively in the first 3 months after injury if they had a preinjury psychiatric disorder or poorer preinjury behavioral adjustment.[9,30] Children with mild TBI are more likely than orthopedic injured controls to show transient or persistent increases in postconcussive symptoms in the first 12 months after injury, especially if the injury was serious.[15,31] Postconcussive symptoms were unrelated to the apolipoprotein epsilon 4 allele.[32] The families of children with mild TBI experienced more distress and burden than the families of orthopedic control children, and this was closely linked with postconcussive symptoms.[33]

The links between family function and psychiatric and/or behavioral function in children with mild to severe TBI are close. Family outcome is typically associated with lower preinjury family function, presence of NPD, more stressors, and use of fewer sources of support.[33-39]

Specific Psychiatric Disorders/Symptom Clusters

Table 1 provides a summary of lesion-behavior correlates for NPDs and postinjury symptom clusters.

Personality Change due to TBI

The most common NPD after severe TBI is personality change due to TBI (PC).[40,41] PC is not a personality disorder. The diagnosis is made in the context of clinically significant symptoms of affective instability, aggression, disinhibited behavior, apathy, or paranoia reasonably judged to be caused by the injury. The Neuropsychiatric Rating Schedule[42] can reliably and validly guide the clinician to justify a diagnosis of PC. Approximately 40% of consecutively hospitalized children with severe TBI had ongoing persistent PC an average of 2 years after the injury.[40] An additional approximately 20% had a history of a remitted and more transient PC. PC occurred in 5% of

Table 1
Lesion-psychiatric correlates after pediatric TBI

Disorder	Lesion Correlate (Timing of Outcome)	Reference
NPD	Lower fractional anisotropy in bilateral frontal, temporal lobes, uncinate fasiculi, centrum semiovale (3 mo)	[12]
PC due to TBI	Superior frontal gyrus (6 and 12 mo)	[10,43]
	Frontal white matter (24 mo)	[43]
ADHD	Right putamen, thalamus (12 mo)	[20,51]
	Orbital frontal gyrus (6 mo)	[46]
PTSD (reexperiencing criterion)	Right limbic area (including cingulum, hippocampus) lower lesion fraction (12 mo)	[63]
PTSD (hyperarousal symptoms)	Left temporal lesions and lower frequency of orbitofrontal lesions (12 mo)	[64]
Obsessions	Mesial prefrontal and temporal (12 mo)	[67]
Obsessive compulsive disorder	Frontal and temporal lobe (3–9 mo)	[66]
Anxiety disorder/subclinical anxiety disorder	Superior frontal gyrus (6 mo) Lower frequency of orbitofrontal lesions (12 mo)	[64,68]
Nonanxious depressive disorder/ subclinical depressive disorder	Left inferior frontal gyrus and left temporal tip (6 mo)	[72]
Anxious depressive disorder/ subclinical depressive disorder	Right frontal lobe white matter and left parietal lobe (6 mo)	[72]
Mania/hypomania	Frontal lobe and temporal lobe (3–24 mo)	[70]

mild/moderate TBI but was always transient. The affective instability, aggressive, and disinhibited subtypes are common, whereas the apathetic and paranoid subtypes are not common.[40,41] Severity of injury is a significant predictor of PC in the first 2 years after TBI.[10,40,41,43] More specifically, PC is associated with superior frontal gyrus lesions in the first year.[10,43] This lesion correlate is consistent with prevailing models of affective regulation implicating the dorsal prefrontal cortex.[44] In the second postinjury year, PC was significantly associated with frontal white matter lesions and preinjury adaptive function.[43] This suggests that although affective regulation problems, associated initially with superior frontal lesions, decrease as other cortical areas subsume this function, subcortical network damage (lesioned white matter tracts) limits eventual recovery. For the purposes of explanation, a mechanistic computer analogy is useful. The analogy is of a motherboard (representing cortex) and a wired network (representing a white matter network) that posit acceptable performance (appropriate affective regulation) with a motherboard replacement if that were the problem but not if the network was damaged. Furthermore, these findings suggest that, similar to the idea of preinjury cognitive reserve,[45] preinjury functional reserve, such as higher preinjury adaptive function, predicts whether a child will have PC persisting through the second postinjury year. The later emergence of preinjury adaptive function as a correlate of PC can be understood through the metaphor of TBI as an avalanche and the individual as a structure that is covered by the avalanche. If the structure is covered but not destroyed by the snow, then, with the passage of time and the melting of the snow pack, the tallest structures (ie, higher premorbid function) emerges (restore function) earlier. If the structure was destroyed, then whatever factors led originally to the structure being among the tallest (eg, genetics to environmental influences) are operational in rebuilding the structure quickest. PC is also associated with a concurrent diagnosis of secondary ADHD and adaptive and intellectual functioning decrements, but is not related to any psychosocial adversity variables.[40] PC tends to be the most debilitating psychiatric syndrome even when comorbid with other NPDs such as ADHD or oppositional defiant disorder (ODD).

VIGNETTE 1

An 11-year-old boy with a severe TBI with preinjury ADHD and ODD had clinically significant moderate irritability (not caused by brain damage) before the injury. After the injury and for 12 months he experienced significant worsening of his irritability. There were no major psychosocial stressors and his academic program was well suited to his abilities. A significant component of his affective instability was attributed to brain injury and therefore he was diagnosed with PC, affective instability subtype.

Secondary ADHD

Secondary ADHD (SADHD) refers to ADHD that develops after TBI. The phenomenology of SADHD includes all ADHD subtypes.[46] SADHD is related to increasing severity of injury and intellectual function, memory, and adaptive function deficits as well as family dysfunction in samples of mild to severe TBI. When study cohorts are limited to severe or to severe/moderate TBI, adaptive deficits are still evident but findings regarding intellectual function outcome are mixed.[20,47] Poorer preinjury family function and greater premorbid psychosocial adversity is associated with postinjury ADHD symptoms and SADHD.[20,48,49] Brain correlates of SADHD include right putamen or thalamic lesions,[50,51] and orbital frontal gyrus lesions.[46] These anatomic findings suggest that lesions in varied locations along specific cortico-striatal-pallidal-thalamic loops may generate a clinical syndrome of SADHD. Neurocognitive studies of SADHD compared with phenotypically overlapping developmental ADHD have been reported but it is too early to reach definitive conclusions regarding their similarities and differences.[49,52–56]

VIGNETTE 2: 2 CASES OF SADHD AND SCHOOL FAILURE

1. *A 12-year old boy with a severe TBI developed SADHD and significant problems with pragmatics of communication. Regulation of anger and sadness was unremarkable. Six months after the injury he was challenged more at school and fell behind his class. He experienced irritability, anger, and sadness, and a diagnosis of an adjustment disorder with mixed emotional features was made. The clinician's formulation was that his affective instability was an indirect result of his TBI; that is, cognitive challenges led ultimately to school failure and his response included irritability and sadness.*

2. *A 13-year old boy with a severe TBI developed SADHD and significant challenges with pragmatics of communication. He was diagnosed with PC, affective instability subtype, because regulation of anger and sadness was impaired in the hospital and persisted throughout the first year after the TBI. Six months after the injury he was challenged more at school and fell behind his class. He became even more irritable and sad but did not meet criteria for a major depression. The clinician's formulation was that his affective instability was a direct result of his TBI; that is, poor mood regulation and cognitive problems led to school failure and reduced his teacher's effectiveness in working with him.*

ODD/Conduct Disorder

New-onset ODD and conduct disorder were reported to occur in 9% and 8% respectively of youth followed for 1 year after admission to a rehabilitation center.[57] The disorders/symptoms were associated with preinjury psychosocial adversity and concurrent symptoms of emotional lability. In a consecutively hospitalized sample of mild-severe TBI, ODD symptoms in the first 12-months after TBI were similarly related to social class, preinjury family function, and preinjury ODD symptoms.[58] Greater severity of TBI predicted ODD symptoms 2 years after injury. Socioeconomic status influenced change (from before TBI) in ODD symptoms at 6, 12, and 24 months after TBI. Only at 2 years after injury was severity of injury a predictor of change in ODD symptoms. A report from a brain injury clinic sample showed that children who developed novel ODD/conduct disorder, compared with children without a lifetime history of the disorder, had significantly more family dysfunction, showed a trend toward a family history of alcohol dependence/abuse, and had milder TBIs.[59] None of the studies of novel ODD/conduct disorder had orthopedic injury controls.

PTSD

PTSD and subsyndromal posttraumatic stress disturbances occur despite neurogenic amnesia. Rates of novel PTSD range from 4% to 13%, although the presence of PTSD symptoms are common (68%) in the first weeks after injury and decline (12%) by 2 year after injury.[60,61] Studies have shown significant predictors and/or correlates of PTSD symptoms to include preinjury mood or anxiety disorder/symptoms, greater injury severity, female gender, early postinjury anxiety and depression symptoms, preinjury psychosocial adversity, and nonanxiety psychiatric diagnoses.[60–62] An imaging study found that the PTSD criterion for reexperiencing was associated with a lower lesion fraction (volumetric fraction of a predefined atlas structure that overlapped with the participant's lesion) in the right limbic area, specifically the cingulum and hippocampus. The right limbic region is frequently activated in functional imaging studies of reexperiencing symptoms in PTSD.[63] In addition, PTSD hyperarousal symptoms were associated with left temporal lesions and absence of left orbitofrontal lesions.[64]

VIGNETTE 3

A 16-year old girl was struck on the right temporal area by a discus thrown by a peer from 9 m (30 feet) away. She experienced about 10 seconds of loss of consciousness and was seen in the emergency room and discharged. Imaging studies including magnetic resonance imaging 18 months after the injury were normal. Over the course of a few weeks she developed a fear of flying objects, which expanded to include not only a discus but any ball kicked or thrown on a sports field, and she became fearful that the vehicle in which she was traveling would be hit by another vehicle. These fears were associated with a full range of PTSD reexperiencing symptoms, avoidance behaviors, and increased arousal. She developed a major depressive disorder with no suicidality. She was irritable but this seemed consistent with and fully accounted for by PTSD and major depression, and therefore PC, affective instability subtype, was not diagnosed. Only with intense effort was she able to maintain her preinjury grades, and she had a full range of inattentive symptoms and met criteria for a provisional diagnosis of ADHD, inattentive type. The diagnosis was provisional because it was unclear whether her inattention could be completely explained by her PTSD and major depression diagnoses. She also developed daily headaches that were partially responsive to low-dose amitriptyline. She had a first-degree relative with panic disorder. She presented for treatment 18-months after the injury and responded well to cognitive behavior therapy and a selective serotonin reuptake inhibitor (SSRI) but had to be strongly encouraged to expose herself to feared situations, including driving. She did not require treatment of ADHD because symptoms resolved entirely with her treatment of PTSD and major depression.

Other Anxiety Disorders

Novel obsessive compulsive disorder occurs following TBI in adolescence.[65,66] Frontal and temporal lobe lesions can precipitate the syndrome in the absence of obvious striatal injury.[66] New onset of obsessions is associated with female gender, psychosocial adversity, and mesial frontal and temporal lesions.[67] A wide variety of other anxiety disorders have been documented after childhood TBI, including overanxious disorder, specific phobia, separation anxiety disorder, and avoidant disorder.[9,21,22] Preinjury anxiety symptoms and younger age at injury correlated positively with postinjury anxiety symptoms.[65] Furthermore, severity of brain injury and postinjury level of stress have been associated with mood/anxiety disorders.[27] Lesions of the superior frontal gyrus were significantly associated with postinjury anxiety symptoms[68] whereas orbitofrontal lesions were associated with fewer anxiety symptoms.[64]

Mania/Hypomania

There are several published case reports on the development of mania or hypomania after childhood TBI.[69] Four of 50 children (8%) from a prospective study of consecutive children hospitalized following TBI developed mania or hypomania.[70] The phenomenology regarding the overlapping diagnoses of mania, PC, and ADHD must be considered in differential diagnosis.[40] Greater severity of injury, frontal and temporal lobe lesions, and family history of mood disorder may be implicated in the cause of mania/hypomania secondary to TBI. Long-lasting episodes and similar frequency of irritability and elation may be typical.[70]

Depressive Disorders

In a retrospective psychiatric interview study,[21] one-quarter of children with severe TBI had an ongoing depressive disorder and one-third of the children had a depressive disorder at some point after the injury. TBI increased the risk of depressive symptoms especially among more socially disadvantaged children, and the depressive symptoms were weakly related to postinjury neurocognitive performance.[71] New-onset depression including disorders with no comorbid new anxiety disorder (nonanxious depression) and disorders with a comorbid new anxiety disorder (anxious depression) was related to left-sided and right-sided lesions and older age at injury compared with children who did not develop depression. Nonanxious depression was associated with left hemisphere lesions specifically in the left inferior frontal gyrus and temporal tip, whereas anxious depression was associated with right hemisphere lesions, specifically in the right frontal lobe white matter, and also left parietal lobe lesions.[72] The association of nonanxious depression with left lesions and anxious depression predominantly with right lesions is similar to adult TBI findings.[73] Anxious depression was also associated with PC and a family history of anxiety disorder.[72]

Psychosis and Autism

There have been only 2 cases of new-onset nonaffective psychosis reported in 6 studies of consecutive admissions of children with TBI that used standardized psychiatric interviews.[8,11,21,22,28,43] However, there has been interest in the possibility that early TBI increases the risk of psychosis in adult life.[74,75] Autism after childhood TBI has not been described, although other forms of brain injury have been implicated in the new onset of autism in childhood (eg, brain tumors).[76] It is important for clinicians to differentiate autism from the qualitatively different disturbances of pragmatic communication and social communication that can be complications of severe TBI in young children.[77,78]

TREATMENT
Nonpharmacologic Treatment Strategies
School
Academic functioning at school corresponds with occupational functioning for adults. Children, especially those with more serious TBI, are the beneficiaries of mandated

services under the Individuals with Disabilities Education Act. Special education ser-vices target poor academic function related to (1) skill deficits in arithmetic, spelling, and reading; (2) emotional and behavioral disorders; or (3) a combination of these skill deficits and emotional and behavioral disorders with or without underlying difficulties of preinjury developmental learning problems in some children. For a more in-depth review of educational and related neuropsychological aspects of pediatric TBI, see Refs.[79,80]

Family-based treatment

One research laboratory is producing a growing body of pediatric TBI literature including randomized controlled trials involving Web-based family and teen problem-solving psychological therapies targeting behavioral problems rather than specific psychiatric disorders.[81–86] The research team's most recent therapeutic refinement is termed counselor-assisted problem solving (CAPS), which is a 6-month Web-based, family-centered intervention that focuses on problem solving, communi-cation, and self-regulation.[82] After an initial in-person session with a therapist, follow-up sessions with the therapist are conducted via Skype. These sessions proceed according to a prearranged standard plan with specific content and the treatment pro-gram is flexible in that supplementary sessions may be provided with content designed to address particular residual problems and needs of each family. Further-more, the CAPS treatment arm provides access to a CAPS Web site that has self-directed didactic content regarding problem-solving skills, video clips modeling these skills, and exercises to practice the skills. The control group in the studies is an Internet resource comparison (IRC) that involves the family and/or teen having access to key Web sites that provide self-directed didactic information about brain injury as well as modules about problem solving around common issues, working with schools, and managing stress.[82] Among the positive results reported for CAPS is an improve-ment in parent-rated behavioral executive functioning in their children,[82] an effect that is greater in the context of lower verbal intelligence of the children.[81] Furthermore, among older adolescents, CAPS was associated with greater improvement in multiple dimensions of externalizing behavior problems compared with IRC. The same research team earlier published on a treatment called teen online problem solving (TOPS), which seems to be closely related to CAPS. Compared with IRC, TOPS has been effective in improving problem solving and depressive symptoms in parents, especially those with low incomes.[85] TOPS resulted in improvement in parent-teen conflict generally and in parent and self-reported teen behavior problems, particularly in adolescents with severe TBI.[84]

Other approaches to treatment include cognitive behavior therapy and restructuring the child's environment to maximize behavioral supports.[80] In addition, training parents to be more effective advocates for the child within the school system can be helpful.[87]

Pharmacotherapies

The reader is referred to a recent comprehensive, albeit bleak, review of neurophar-macology of pediatric brain injury.[88] In contrast with the promising developments in nonpharmacologic treatment strategies, that review concludes that evidence support-ing the off-label use of numerous agents for children with TBI is limited or nonexistent.

PC due to TBI: Labile and Aggressive Subtypes

In the absence of treatment studies of children with PC, the following anecdotal guidelines are offered. The labile and aggressive types frequently co-occur[41] and respond similarly to treatment. Mood-stabilizing anticonvulsants such as carbamaz-epine and valproic acid can be effective when combined with a behavior modification program targeting aggressive behavior. The addition of an SSRI can yield additional benefit.

PC due to TBI: Disinhibited, Paranoid, Apathetic Subtypes

The disinhibited subtype is difficult to treat pharmacologically or behaviorally. The paranoid subtype is rare. Use of neuroleptic medication such as ziprasidone may be helpful in the acute hospitalization or rehabilitation unit if the child or adolescent is agitated or paranoid and the symptoms are impeding compliance with treatment regimens.[89] The potential risks from neuroleptics with regard to aberrations in neuronal recovery have been described in animal models.[90] The rare apathetic sub-type may respond to stimulant medication or SSRIs.

There may be episodes when the child has intense lability, aggression, hyperactiv-ity, and inattention, and meets criteria for overlapping syndromes of PC, mania or hypomania, and ADHD.[9] Mood stabilizers may help and stimulants are not necessarily contraindicated.[91]

ADHD

Several reports of stimulants administered to children with TBI who have attention and concentration deficits show positive results, although the data are mixed.[92] Anecdotal evidence from the author's practice suggests that children diagnosed with SADHD respond to stimulant medication. There have been no studies of bupropion or tricyclic antidepressant medication for SADHD. The use of bupropion is avoided because of the risk of seizures. Caution should be observed when prescribing the tricyclic antide-pressants because of cardiac conduction side effects.

Depression

There are no treatment studies of depressive disorders after pediatric TBI. Clinical experience suggests that SSRIs are effective.[93]

Emerging Treatment Approaches

Pharmacologic research has been impeded by the difficulty in identifying and enrolling a sufficient number of children and adolescents with TBI with the same NPD at any single research site. Multicenter collaborations exemplified by the methodology of the Children's Oncology Group have been suggested to address the problem.[88] Expansion of the mission of existing research units in pediatric psychopharmacology to include multisite medication trials related to NPDs would rapidly advance the knowl-edge base. A related potential solution to this challenge has been initiated by means of a single patient trial–published protocol across multiple sites for stimulant treatment of SADHD.[94]

Advances in psychotherapy research for children and adolescents with TBI will include testing of treatment modalities that have been proved effective for behavioral, emotional, or family problems in uninjured populations. An example of an established treatment that may emerge as a treatment of a TBI cohort includes parent-child inter-action therapy.[95]

The most important ongoing and emerging intervention strategies involve preven-tion of injury. Education with regard to the use of bicycle helmets, enhancing motor vehicle safety, decreasing alcohol-related motor vehicle accidents, and decreasing the risk of child abuse and neglect are some of the methods to prevent or attenuate the morbidity caused by pediatric TBI.[96]

SUMMARY

Pediatric TBI is a major public health problem. The psychiatrist has a central role in working with affected children and adolescents because psychiatric disorders are common both before and after injury. There is a close relationship between psychiatric disorders and family function. NPDs are associated with specific injury and psychosocial variables, including family dysfunction, which can be measured soon after injury. This association allows the potential recognition of children who are at high risk for psychiatric problems before they emerge. The categorization of behavioral complications of TBI into psychiatric syndromes permits a logical pharmacologic and psychological treatment approach. Pharmacologic research for NPDs is negligible, whereas psychotherapy research is showing promise in the treatment of common domains of behavior such as self-regulation, communication, and aspects of family function, but not specifically for NPDs. Cognitive function impairments complicate school reentry and limit educational achievement. When cognitive function deficits are associated with psychiatric problems management is particularly challenging. Additional biologic research, such as with gene expression methodology, advanced imaging modalities such as magnetoencephalography and diffusion spectrum imaging, as well as psychosocial research on injury risk and psychiatric outcome, is necessary for promotion of effective primary and secondary prevention of behavioral morbidity.

REFERENCES

1. Langlois JA, Rutland-Brown W, Thomas KE. The incidence of traumatic brain injury among children in the United States: differences by race. J Head Trauma Rehabil 2005;20(3):229–38.
2. Kraus JF, Rock A, Hemyari P. Brain injuries among infants, children, adolescents, and young adults. Am J Dis Child 1990;144(6):684–91.
3. Levin HS, Aldrich EF, Saydjari C, et al. Severe head injury in children: experience of the Traumatic Coma Data Bank. Neurosurgery 1992;31(3):435–43 [discussion: 443–4].
4. Levin HS, Culhane KA, Mendelsohn D, et al. Cognition in relation to magnetic resonance imaging in head-injured children and adolescents. Arch Neurol 1993;50(9):897–905.
5. Kochanek PM. Pediatric traumatic brain injury: quo vadis? Dev Neurosci 2006; 28(4–5):244–55.
6. Kochanek PM, Bell MJ, Bayir H. Quo vadis 2010? - carpe diem: challenges and opportunities in pediatric traumatic brain injury. Dev Neurosci 2010;32(5–6):335–42.
7. Asarnow RF, Satz P, Light R, et al. Behavior problems and adaptive functioning in children with mild and severe closed head injury. J Pediatr Psychol 1991; 16(5):543–55.
8. Brown G, Chadwick O, Shaffer D, et al. A prospective study of children with head injuries: III. Psychiatric sequelae. Psychol Med 1981;11(1):63–78.
9. Max JE, Smith WL Jr, Sato Y, et al. Traumatic brain injury in children and adolescents: psychiatric disorders in the first three months. J Am Acad Child Adolesc Psychiatry 1997;36(1):94–102.
10. Max JE, Levin HS, Landis J, et al. Predictors of personality change due to traumatic brain injury in children and adolescents in the first six months after injury. J Am Acad Child Adolesc Psychiatry 2005;44(5):434–42.
11. Max JE, Wilde EA, Bigler ED, et al. Psychiatric disorders after pediatric traumatic brain injury: a prospective, longitudinal, controlled study. J Neuropsychiatry Clin Neurosci 2012;24(4):427–36.

12. Max JE, Wilde EA, Bigler ED, et al. Neuroimaging correlates of novel psychiatric disorders after pediatric traumatic brain injury. J Am Acad Child Adolesc Psychiatry 2012;51(11):1208–17.

13. Fletcher JM, Ewing-Cobbs L, Miner ME, et al. Behavioral changes after closed head injury in children. J Consult Clin Psychol 1990;58(1):93–8.

14. Rivara JM, Jaffe KM, Polissar NL, et al. Predictors of family functioning and change 3 years after traumatic brain injury in children. Arch Phys Med Rehabil 1996;77(8):754–64.

15. Yeates KO, Taylor HG, Rusin J, et al. Longitudinal trajectories of postconcussive symptoms in children with mild traumatic brain injuries and their relationship to acute clinical status. Pediatrics 2009;123(3):735–43.

16. Kurowski BG, Taylor HG, Yeates KO, et al. Caregiver ratings of long-term executive dysfunction and attention problems after early childhood traumatic brain injury: family functioning is important. PM R 2011;3(9):836–45.

17. Yeates KO, Armstrong K, Janusz J, et al. Long-term attention problems in children with traumatic brain injury. J Am Acad Child Adolesc Psychiatry 2005; 44(6):574–84.

18. Ewing-Cobbs L, Prasad MR, Kramer L, et al. Late intellectual and academic outcomes following traumatic brain injury sustained during early childhood. J Neurosurg 2006;105(Suppl 4):287–96.

19. Bijur P, Golding J, Haslum M, et al. Behavioral predictors of injury in school-age children. Am J Dis Child 1988;142(12):1307–12.

20. Gerring JP, Brady KD, Chen A, et al. Premorbid prevalence of ADHD and development of secondary ADHD after closed head injury. J Am Acad Child Adolesc Psychiatry 1998;37(6):647–54.

21. Max JE, Koele SL, Smith WL Jr, et al. Psychiatric disorders in children and adolescents after severe traumatic brain injury: a controlled study. J Am Acad Child Adolesc Psychiatry 1998;37(8):832–40.

22. Max JE, Robin DA, Lindgren SD, et al. Traumatic brain injury in children and adolescents: psychiatric disorders at two years. J Am Acad Child Adolesc Psychiatry 1997;36(9):1278–85.

23. Massagli TL, Fann JR, Burington BE, et al. Psychiatric illness after mild traumatic brain injury in children. Arch Phys Med Rehabil 2004;85:1428–34.

24. Rune V. Acute head injuries in children. A retrospective epidemiologic, child psychiatric and electroencephalographic study on primary school children in Umea. Acta Paediatr Scand Suppl 1970;209(Suppl):3–12.

25. Max JE, Dunisch DL. Traumatic brain injury in a child psychiatry outpatient clinic: a controlled study. J Am Acad Child Adolesc Psychiatry 1997;36(3):404–11.

26. Max JE, Schachar RJ, Landis J, et al. Psychiatric disorders in children and adolescents in the first six months after mild traumatic brain injury. J Neuropsychiatry Clin Neurosci 2013;25(3):187–97.

27. Luis CA, Mittenberg W. Mood and anxiety disorders following pediatric traumatic brain injury: a prospective study. J Clin Exp Neuropsychol 2002;24(3):270–9.

28. Lehmkuhl G, Thoma W. Development in children after severe head injury. In: Rothenberger A, editor. Brain and behavior in child psychiatry. Berlin: Springer-Verlag; 1990. p. 267–82.

29. McKinlay A, Dalrymple-Alford JC, Horwood LJ, et al. Long term psychosocial outcomes after mild head injury in early childhood. J Neurol Neurosurg Psychiatr 2002;73(3):281–8.

30. Yeates KO, Luria J, Bartkowski H, et al. Postconcussive symptoms in children with mild closed head injuries. J Head Trauma Rehabil 1999;14(4):337–50.

31. Yeates KO, Kaizar E, Rusin J, et al. Reliable change in postconcussive symptoms and its functional consequences among children with mild traumatic brain injury. Arch Pediatr Adolesc Med 2012;166(7):615–22.

32. Moran LM, Taylor HG, Ganesaligam K, et al. Apolipoprotein E4 as a predictor of outcomes in pediatric mild traumatic brain injury. J Neurotrauma 2009;26(9): 1489–95.

33. Ganesalingam K, Yeates KO, Ginn MS, et al. Family burden and parental distress following mild traumatic brain injury in children and its relationship to post-concussive symptoms. J Pediatr Psychol 2008;33(6):621–9.

34. Taylor HG, Yeates KO, Wade SL, et al. Influences on first-year recovery from traumatic brain injury in children. Neuropsychology 1999;13(1):76–89.

35. Yeates KO, Taylor HG, Drotar D, et al. Preinjury family environment as a determinant of recovery from traumatic brain injuries in school-age children. J Int Neuropsychol Soc 1997;3(6):617–30.

36. Max JE, Castillo CS, Robin DA, et al. Predictors of family functioning after traumatic brain injury in children and adolescents. J Am Acad Child Adolesc Psychiatry 1998;37(1):83–90.

37. Josie KL, Peterson CC, Burant C, et al. Predicting family burden following childhood traumatic brain injury: a cumulative risk approach. J Head Trauma Rehabil 2008;23(6):357–68.

38. Rivara JB, Jaffe KM, Fay GC, et al. Family functioning and injury severity as predictors of child functioning one year following traumatic brain injury. Arch Phys Med Rehabil 1993;74(10):1047–55.

39. Taylor HG, Yeates KO, Wade SL, et al. Bidirectional child-family influences on outcomes of traumatic brain injury in children. J Int Neuropsychol Soc 2001; 7(6):755–67.

40. Max JE, Koele SL, Castillo CC, et al. Personality change disorder in children and adolescents following traumatic brain injury. J Int Neuropsychol Soc 2000;6(3): 279–89.

41. Max JE, Robertson BA, Lansing AE. The phenomenology of personality change due to traumatic brain injury in children and adolescents. J Neuropsychiatry Clin Neurosci 2001;13(2):161–70.

42. Max JE, Castillo CS, Lindgren SD, et al. The Neuropsychiatric Rating Schedule: reliability and validity. J Am Acad Child Adolesc Psychiatry 1998;37(3):297–304.

43. Max JE, Levin HS, Schachar RJ, et al. Predictors of personality change due to traumatic brain injury in children and adolescents six to twenty-four months after injury. J Neuropsychiatry Clin Neurosci 2006;18(1):21–32.

44. Mayberg HS. Limbic-cortical dysregulation: a proposed model of depression. J Neuropsychiatry Clin Neurosci 1997;9(3):471–81.

45. Kesler SR, Adams HF, Blasey CM, et al. Premorbid intellectual functioning, education, and brain size in traumatic brain injury: an investigation of the cognitive reserve hypothesis. Appl Neuropsychol 2003;10(3):153–62.

46. Max JE, Schachar RJ, Levin HS, et al. Predictors of attention-deficit/ hyperactivity disorder within 6 months after pediatric traumatic brain injury. J Am Acad Child Adolesc Psychiatry 2005;44(10):1032–40.

47. Max JE, Lansing AE, Koele SL, et al. Attention deficit hyperactivity disorder in children and adolescents following traumatic brain injury. Dev Neuropsychol 2004;25(1–2):159–77.

48. Max JE, Arndt S, Castillo CS, et al. Attention-deficit hyperactivity symptomatology after traumatic brain injury: a prospective study. J Am Acad Child Adolesc Psychiatry 1998;37(8):841–7.

49. Slomine BS, Salorio CF, Grados MA, et al. Differences in attention, executive functioning, and memory in children with and without ADHD after severe traumatic brain injury. J Int Neuropsychol Soc 2005;11(5):645–53.
50. Gerring J, Brandy K, Chen A, et al. Neuroimaging variables related to development of secondary attention deficit hyperactivity disorder after closed head injury in children and adolescents. Brain Inj 2000;14(3):205–18.
51. Herskovits EH, Megalooikonomou V, Davatzikos C, et al. Is the spatial distribution of brain lesions associated with closed-head injury predictive of subsequent development of attention-deficit/hyperactivity disorder? Analysis with brain-image database. Radiology 1999;213(2):389–94.
52. Schachar R, Levin HS, Max JE, et al. Attention deficit hyperactivity disorder symptoms and response inhibition after closed head injury in children: do pre-injury behavior and injury severity predict outcome? Dev Neuropsychol 2004; 25(1–2):179–98.
53. Ornstein TJ, Max JE, Schachar R, et al. Response inhibition in children with and without ADHD after traumatic brain injury. J Neuropsychol 2013;7(1):1–11.
54. Sinopoli KJ, Schachar R, Dennis M. Traumatic brain injury and secondary attention-deficit/hyperactivity disorder in children and adolescents: the effect of reward on inhibitory control. J Clin Exp Neuropsychol 2011;33(7):805–19.
55. Wassenberg R, Max JE, Lindgren SD, et al. Sustained attention in children and adolescents after traumatic brain injury: relation to severity of injury, adaptive functioning, ADHD and social background. Brain Inj 2004;18(8):751–64.
56. Dennis M, Sinopoli KJ, Fletcher JM, et al. Puppets, robots, critics, and actors within a taxonomy of attention for developmental disorders. J Int Neuropsychol Soc 2008;14(5):673–90.
57. Gerring JP, Grados MA, Slomine B, et al. Disruptive behaviour disorders and disruptive symptoms after severe paediatric traumatic brain injury. Brain Inj 2009;23(12):944–55.
58. Max JE, Castillo CS, Bokura H, et al. Oppositional defiant disorder symptomatology after traumatic brain injury: a prospective study. J Nerv Ment Dis 1998;186(6):325–32.
59. Max JE, Lindgren SD, Knutson C, et al. Child and adolescent traumatic brain injury: correlates of disruptive behavior disorders. Brain Inj 1998;12(1):41–52.
60. Max JE, Castillo CS, Robin DA, et al. Posttraumatic stress symptomatology after childhood traumatic brain injury. J Nerv Ment Dis 1998;186:589–96.
61. Gerring JP, Slomine B, Vasa RA, et al. Clinical predictors of posttraumatic stress disorder after closed head injury in children. J Am Acad Child Adolesc Psychiatry 2002;41(2):157–65.
62. Levi RB, Drotar D, Yeates KO, et al. Posttraumatic stress symptoms in children following orthopedic or traumatic brain injury. J Clin Child Psychol 1999;28(2):232–43.
63. Herskovits EH, Gerring JP, Davatzikos C, et al. Is the spatial distribution of brain lesions associated with closed-head injury in children predictive of subsequent development of posttraumatic stress disorder? Radiology 2002;224(2):345–51.
64. Vasa RA, Grados M, Slomine B, et al. Neuroimaging correlates of anxiety after pediatric traumatic brain injury. Biol Psychiatry 2004;55(3):208–16.
65. Vasa RA, Gerring JP, Grados M, et al. Anxiety after severe pediatric closed head injury. J Am Acad Child Adolesc Psychiatry 2002;41(2):148–56.
66. Max JE, Smith WL Jr, Lindgren SD, et al. Case study: obsessive-compulsive disorder after severe traumatic brain injury in an adolescent. J Am Acad Child Adolesc Psychiatry 1995;34(1):45–9.

67. Grados MA, Vasa RA, Riddle MA, et al. New onset obsessive-compulsive symptoms in children and adolescents with severe traumatic brain injury. Depress Anxiety 2008;25(5):398–407.
68. Max JE, Keatley E, Wilde EA, et al. Anxiety disorders in children and adolescents in the first six months after traumatic brain injury. J Neuropsychiatry Clin Neurosci 2011;23(1):29–39.
69. Sayal K, Ford T, Pipe R. Bipolar disorder after head injury. J Am Acad Child Adolesc Psychiatry 2000;39(4):525–8.
70. Max JE, Smith WL, Sato Y, et al. Mania and hypomania following traumatic brain injury in children and adolescents. Neurocase 1997;3:119–26.
71. Kirkwood M, Janusz J, Yeates KO, et al. Prevalence and correlates of depressive symptoms following traumatic brain injuries in children. Child Neuropsychol 2000;6(3):195–208.
72. Max JE, Keatley E, Wilde EA, et al. Depression in children and adolescents in the first 6 months after traumatic brain injury. Int J Dev Neurosci 2012;30(3):239–45.
73. Jorge RE, Robinson RG, Starkstein SE, et al. Depression and anxiety following traumatic brain injury. J Neuropsychiatry Clin Neurosci 1993;5(4):369–74.
74. Wilcox JA, Nasrallah HA. Childhood head trauma and psychosis. Psychiatry Res 1987;21(4):303–6.
75. Malaspina D, Goetz RR, Friedman JH, et al. Traumatic brain injury and schizophrenia in members of schizophrenia and bipolar disorder pedigrees. Am J Psychiatry 2001;158(3):440–6.
76. Hoon AH, Reiss AL. The mesial-temporal lobe and autism: case report and review. Dev Med Child Neurol 1992;34(3):252–9.
77. Ewing-Cobbs L, Prasad MR, Swank P, et al. Social communication in young children with traumatic brain injury: relations with corpus callosum morphometry. Int J Dev Neurosci 2012;30(3):247–54.
78. Dennis M, Purvis K, Barnes MA, et al. Understanding of literal truth, ironic criticism, and deceptive praise following childhood head injury. Brain Lang 2001;78(1):1–16.
79. Max JE, Ibrahim F, Levin H. Neuropsychological and psychiatric outcomes of traumatic brain injury in children. In: Nass RD, Frank Y, editors. Cognitive and behavioral abnormalities of pediatric diseases. New York: Oxford University Press; 2010. p. 647–59.
80. Ylvisaker M, Turkstra L, Coehlo C, et al. Behavioural interventions for children and adults with behaviour disorders after TBI: a systematic review of the evidence. Brain Inj 2007;21(8):769–805.
81. Karver CL, Wade SL, Cassedy A, et al. Cognitive reserve as a moderator of responsiveness to an online problem-solving intervention for adolescents with complicated mild-to-severe traumatic brain injury. Child Neuropsychol 2013. [Epub ahead of print].
82. Kurowski BG, Wade SL, Kirkwood MW, et al. Online problem-solving therapy for executive dysfunction after child traumatic brain injury. Pediatrics 2013;132(1):e158–66.
83. Wade SL, Stancin T, Kirkwood M, et al. Counselor-assisted problem solving (CAPS) improves behavioral outcomes in older adolescents with complicated mild to severe TBI. J Head Trauma Rehabil 2013. [Epub ahead of print].
84. Wade SL, Walz NC, Carey J, et al. Effect on behavior problems of teen online problem-solving for adolescent traumatic brain injury. Pediatrics 2011;128(4):e947–53.

85. Wade SL, Walz NC, Carey J, et al. A randomized trial of teen online problem solving: efficacy in improving caregiver outcomes after brain injury. Health Psychol 2012;31(6):767–76.

86. Wade SL, Walz NC, Carey J, et al. A randomized trial of teen online problem solving for improving executive function deficits following pediatric traumatic brain injury. J Head Trauma Rehabil 2010;25(6):409–15.

87. Glang A, McLaughlin K, Schroeder S. Using interactive multimedia to teach parent advocacy skills: an exploratory study. J Head Trauma Rehabil 2007; 22(3):198–205.

88. Pangilinan PH, Giacoletti-Argento A, Shellhaas R, et al. Neuropharmacology in pediatric brain injury: a review. PM R 2010;2(12):1127–40.

89. Scott LK, Green R, McCarthy PJ, et al. Agitation and/or aggression after traumatic brain injury in the pediatric population treated with ziprasidone. Clinical article. J Neurosurg Pediatr 2009;3(6):484–7.

90. Kline AE, Hoffman AN, Cheng JP, et al. Chronic administration of antipsychotics impede behavioral recovery after experimental traumatic brain injury. Neurosci Lett 2008;448(3):263–7.

91. Max JE, Richards L, Hamdan-Allen G. Case study: antimanic effectiveness of dextroamphetamine in a brain-injured adolescent. J Am Acad Child Adolesc Psychiatry 1995;34(4):472–6.

92. Jin C, Schachar R. Methylphenidate treatment of attention-deficit/hyperactivity disorder secondary to traumatic brain injury: a critical appraisal of treatment studies. CNS Spectr 2004;9(3):217–26.

93. Warden DL, Gordon B, McAllister TW, et al. Guidelines for the pharmacologic treatment of neurobehavioral sequelae of traumatic brain injury. J Neurotrauma 2006;23(10):1468–501.

94. Senior HE, McKinlay L, Nikles J, et al. Central nervous system stimulants for secondary attention deficit-hyperactivity disorder after paediatric traumatic brain injury: a rationale and protocol for single patient (n-of-1) multiple cross-over trials. BMC Pediatr 2013;13:89.

95. Cohen ML, Heaton SC, Ginn N, et al. Parent-child interaction therapy as a family-oriented approach to behavioral management following pediatric traumatic brain injury: a case report. J Pediatr Psychol 2012;37(3):251–61.

96. Kraus JF. Epidemiological features of brain injury in children: occurrence, children at risk, causes and manner of injury, severity, and outcomes, in traumatic head injury in children. New York: Oxford University Press; 1995. p. 22–39.

Index

Note: Page numbers of article titles are in **boldface** type.

A

Abulia, 106
Adjustment disorders, depressive disorder *vs.,* 17
Affective lability, characterization of, 35
    evaluation of, 35
    prevalence of, 35
    treatment of, nonpharmacologic, 36
        pharmacologic, 36
Aggression, assessment of, 41–42
    behavioral management techniques for, 42
    characterization of, 40
    cognitive behavioral therapy for, 42
    co-morbidities with, 41
    frequency of, 41
    organic aggressive syndrome and, 40
    as personality change, 133–134
    pharmacotherapy for, 42–43
    typologies of, 40–41
Akinetic mutism, 106
Amantadine, for affective lability, 36
    for depressive disorders, 20
    for disinhibition, 40
    for irritability, 38
Anticonvulsants, for aggression, 43
    for bipolar and related disorders, 23
    for psychosis caused by TBI, 119
Antipsychotics, for acute aggression, 42
    atypical, for bipolar and related disorders, 23–24
    for psychosis caused by TBI, 119
Apathy, correlates of, 107–108
    definition of, 103–104
    diagnosis of, ambulatory actigrapy in, 106
        Children's Motivation Scale in, 105
        criteria for, 104–105
        mental status examination in, 105
        severity rating scales in, 105–106
    differential diagnosis of, 106–107
    frequency of, 107
    mechanism of, arousal system dysfunction in, 108
        imaging studies of, 108
        lesions in, 108

Psychiatr Clin N Am 37 (2014) 141–147
http://dx.doi.org/10.1016/S0193-953X(14)00009-4
0193-953X/14/$ – see front matter © 2014 Elsevier Inc. All rights reserved.

Moving?

Make sure your subscription moves with you!

To notify us of your new address, find your **Clinics Account Number** (located on your mailing label above your name), and contact customer service at:

Email: journalscustomerservice-usa@elsevier.com

800-654-2452 (subscribers in the U.S. & Canada)
314-447-8871 (subscribers outside of the U.S. & Canada)

Fax number: 314-447-8029

Elsevier Health Sciences Division
Subscription Customer Service
3251 Riverport Lane
Maryland Heights, MO 63043

ELSEVIER